GAS GRIDDLE COOKBOOK

Master Easy and Flavorful Recipes
to Elevate Your Grilling and Wow Every Time

Table of Contents

Introduction

If there's one kitchen appliance with the means to revolutionize your cooking game, it's the gas griddle. Though often overlooked in favor of its flashier kitchen cousins, this modest tool is a true kitchen workhorse, capable of churning out restaurant-quality dishes effortlessly. Why sweat over a hot stovetop, juggling multiple pans and spatulas, just to get breakfast on the table? With a gas griddle, you can make pancakes, toast, bacon, and perfectly-cooked eggs all at once.

Between mastering the perfect temperature, figuring out the best cooking techniques, and sorting through the endless recipe options, it's easy to feel overwhelmed here, but that's precisely why you have this book—to take the guesswork out of griddle cooking and become a griddle maestro in your own right.

Unlike other griddle cookbooks that assume prior experience, this one is designed to be accessible, user-friendly, and perfect for beginners and seasoned home cooks. It is your personal griddle coach, here to walk you through every step of the process, from buying your very first gas griddle to comfortably searing, sizzling, and serving. If you've never so much as cracked an egg on a griddle, you'll find everything you need to do just that and plenty more.

Laid out using language that's about as clear as day, there are foolproof recipes, crystal-clear instructions, and gorgeous full-color photos to inspire you. Perhaps most importantly, you'll be inspired to think outside the (griddle) box. Far too often, the griddle is relegated to pancake and breakfast duty, never realizing the full scope of its impressive potential, but that ends right here. Once you master the basics, you'll be shocked by just how versatile a gas griddle can be. Sure, it's a breakfast all-star, but it's also amazing for searing steaks, charring vegetables, warming tortillas, and even baking flatbreads.

Forget about those stressful trial-and-error experiments in the kitchen—Gas Griddle Cookbook has it all covered, from start to delicious finish, no matter what you're cooking, breakfast, lunch, dinner, and everything in between.

Chapter 1:
Getting Started with Your Gas Griddle

Are you tired of the same old routine in the kitchen? Pancakes stuck to the pan, burger buns that won't brown and don't even get started on the dreaded breakfast potato dilemma. If your life in the kitchen has been feeling a little lackluster lately, it might be time to consider an upgrade—and no, not your cooking skills. How would you like to invest in a gas griddle? You might be thinking, "Gas griddles are just for professional chefs, right?" Wrong.

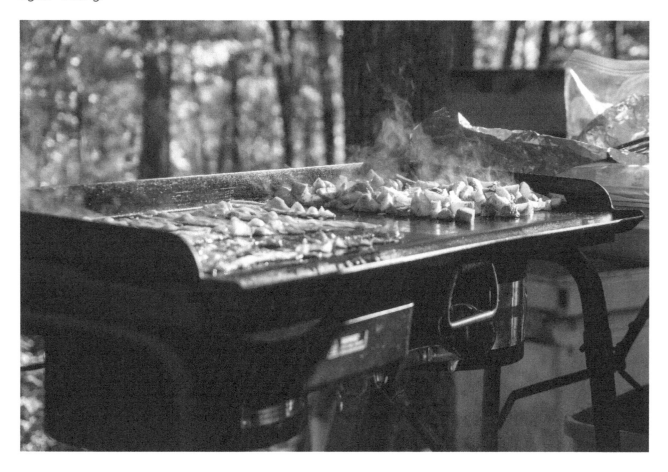

These clever cooktops have recently become increasingly popular in residential kitchens, giving everyday cooks like you a chance to channel your inner Gordon Ramsey and take your meals to the next level.

With all the different types and features available, choosing the right gas griddle can feel a bit much. Should you go for a classic flat-top model, a combo unit with extra functionality, or a compact, portable version? What kind of temperature controls and cooking capacity do you really need? Gas griddles come in all shapes and sizes, and each has its own special set of tricks. Here's a look at some of the most common types and what makes them special:

- **Flat-top Griddles**
  Flat-top gas griddles feature a large, even cooking surface ideal for making pancakes, eggs, burgers, and other foods requiring a flat, heated surface. Think of a well-seasoned cast-iron skillet but way bigger. These griddles usually have adjustable temperature controls for precise heat regulation throughout the cooking area. The smooth, steel cooking surfaces are also easy to clean. Some models

even have grease management systems to collect and dispose of excess fat and oil. Flat-top griddles are available in different sizes to accommodate different cooking volume needs.

- **Combo Griddles**
  Combo gas griddles are do-it-all problem solvers. They combine a flat-top griddle with extra cooking elements, such as grill plates or a built-in fryer. This versatile design allows users to grill, griddle, and fry all on one appliance, cementing it as a go-to pick for both residential and commercial kitchens. The separate temperature controls for each cooking zone provide flexibility, letting you cook many things simultaneously. The space-saving design of combo griddles maximizes cooking capacity in a compact footprint.

- **Portable Griddles**
  Portable gas griddles are a convenient option for cooking on the go, at tailgates, or in tiny kitchens with limited counter space. These lightweight and compact models are designed for easy transport and storage, often featuring foldable or detachable legs for quick setup and breakdown. While the temperature controls may be more basic than in full-size models, portable griddles are still reliable for efficient cooking on disposable propane canisters or by connecting to a larger gas supply. The cooking surface size is generally smaller than stationary griddles, but they are an excellent choice for those who need to cook on the go or when space is at a premium.

Regardless of the specific type, the major things to look for in a gas griddle are even heating, responsive temperature controls, smart grease management, and easy cleanup. Figuring out your cooking needs and available space will help you choose the gas griddle that will be your new best friend in the kitchen.

ESSENTIAL TOOLS AND ACCESSORIES FOR USING A GAS GRIDDLE
Beyond the griddle itself, there are several tools and accessories that you'll need for griddle cooking, including:

- **Spatulas:** Ever tried to flip a pancake with a tiny, flimsy spatula? It's almost always a disaster. The right spatula is important. Look for sturdy, wide spatulas with long, angled handles that can easily slide under your food and maneuver it around the hot griddle surface. Metal spatulas are best since they can withstand high heat without warping or melting.

- **Scrapers:** Cleaning a griddle is sometimes exhausting, but a good scraper makes the job much easier. You'll understand why when you try to scrape off gunky, stuck-on food bits with just a regular old knife. A sharp, beveled-edge scraper glides across the surface, effortlessly clearing away grease and residue between batches, so your griddle is ready to go for the next round.

- **Oil Dispensers:** Drizzling oil onto a hot griddle with an unsteady hand might lead to a messy spill. An oil dispenser lets you evenly coat the surface with just enough oil or cooking fat before heating up. It's a simple tool, but it makes a huge difference in preventing sticking and ensuring even browning of your food.

- **Grill Presses:** Sometimes, you want that signature flat, seared look on your burgers, sandwiches, or other foods. A grill press is a heavy, flat weight used to firmly press down on the items as they cook, giving them that classic diner-style aesthetic and texture.

- **Griddle Covers:** When you're not actively using your gas griddle, you'll want to protect it from dust, debris, and potential damage. A custom-fitted cover functions as a shield, keeping your griddle protected, so it's good to go for your next cooking session.

- **Heat-resistant mitts:** A griddle surface is extremely hot, and handling that with your bare hands is begging for trouble. You don't want to learn that one the hard way. A good set of heat-resistant gloves or mitts is a must-have for safely moving food on and off the griddle.

MAINTAINING YOUR GAS GRIDDLE

Proper cleaning and storage are fundamental to extending the life and performance of your gas griddle. Here's how you can keep your griddle in great shape:

- **Cleaning the Cooking Surface**

  After you're done with your gas griddle, you'll want to give it a good clean. The surface has to cool down completely because you don't want to be scrubbing away at a scorching hot griddle. Once it's a good temperature, grab your griddle scraper and get to work. The sharp edge will quickly scrap off any food bits or grease. Be gentle; you wouldn't want to scratch up that nice cooking surface. Don't use anything too abrasive, like steel wool pads, because they can really do a number on the griddle. Instead, wipe it down with a damp cloth or some paper towels. If you need to give it a more thorough clean, use a small amount of mild dish soap and warm water, but make sure to rinse it all off afterward.

- **Caring for the Exterior**

  The outside of your gas griddle needs to look good too. Wipe it down with a damp cloth to remove any spills or fingerprints. Avoid harsh chemical cleaners because they could discolor or damage the metal. If your griddle has any stainless steel accents, you can use a dedicated stainless steel cleaner to keep that shiny, professional look.

- **Seasoning the Cooking Surface**

  You'll want to give your griddle a little "seasoning" every so often to maintain that slick, nonstick surface. It's easy; just apply a thin layer of cooking oil and heat the griddle to medium–high for 10 to 15 minutes. This will build up a protective coating that will prevent your food from sticking, even for tricky items like pancakes or eggs.

- **Proper Storage**

  When you're done cooking, and the griddle is completely cool, it must be properly stored. Gas griddles should be kept in a well-ventilated area, away from anything that could be a fire hazard. Covering the surface will help keep dust and grime off when it's not in use.

SAFETY TIPS AND TECHNIQUES FOR HANDLING A GRIDDLE

- **Protect Your Hands:** Those metal griddle surfaces can get blazing hot—freshly poured lava hot. Trying to grab a sizzling hot burger with your bare hands could painfully ruin your entire afternoon. Invest in a good pair of heat-resistant gloves or mitts to shield your hands from those intense temperatures.

- **Ventilate before Igniting:** Before you even think about lighting up your gas griddle, open that lid or remove any covers first. This allows the gas to properly vent out, preventing a potential kaboom when you go to ignite it.

- **Use the Igniter, Not the Knob:** Reaching over a closed-up griddle and just turning the control knob to light it is a big no-no. That trapped gas could suddenly ignite and give you one heck of a painful surprise. Use the built-in igniter or a long match to light the burners carefully instead.

- **Keep an Eye on the Flames:** Pay close attention to the height and color of the flames as your griddle heats up. You want nice, steady blue flames, not tall, yellow, flickering ones. Adjust the controls to maintain that even, consistent heat.

- **Extinguish Flare-ups Fast:** If the flames ever start to go crazy and flare up unexpectedly, don't hesitate—immediately turn all the control knobs to the off position.

- **Clean up Spills Quickly:** Griddles get really messy with all that grease and food flying around. Wipe up any spills on the surface right away to prevent potential fires down the line.

- **Empty The Grease Tray:** Let the grease tray overflow, and you're just asking for trouble. Stay on top of regularly emptying it to keep things safe and prevent any dangerous situations.

- **Don't Move a Hot Mess:** Attempting to lug around a hot griddle full of bubbling grease is about as smart as trying to put out a fire with gasoline. Wait until the temperature is cool before attempting to move the unit.

- **Give It Some Space:** When setting up your gas griddle, place it in a well-ventilated area with plenty of clear space around the sides and back. You don't want it crammed into a corner or next to anything flammable.

- **Dress for Success:** Wearing loose, dangling clothing while cooking on a hot griddle is a terrible idea. Stick to close-fitting garments to keep everything tucked away from the flames.

SEASONING YOUR GRIDDLE

Seasoning a brand-new gas griddle might seem like an extra step, but it's worth it for a better experience and durability. Seasoning is the process of creating a thin, protective coating on the cooking surface through the application and heating of cooking oil. This process develops a natural, nonstick surface on the griddle. As the oil polymerizes and bonds to the metal, it fills in microscopic pores and creates a smooth, slick finish. Seasoning also protects the griddle from rust and corrosion. The oil coating becomes a barrier, shielding the metal from moisture and humidity that can cause deterioration.

With that in mind, it's time to walk through the step-by-step process of seasoning a gas griddle for new units and ongoing maintenance.

For a New Unit

- Thoroughly clean the entire cooking surface with mild dish soap and warm water. Rinse and dry completely.
- Apply a thin, even layer of high-heat cooking oil, such as vegetable, canola, or grapeseed oil, over the griddle surface.
- Turn the griddle on to medium-high heat and let it heat up for 15 to 20 minutes. This gives the oil time to polymerize and bond to the metal fully.
- Once the griddle is hot, use a paper towel or clean cloth to wipe away any excess oil carefully. The surface should be left with a subtle, satiny sheen.
- Leave the griddle to cool completely before using it for the first time.

For Maintenance

To maintain your griddle, you'll need to re-season it periodically, especially if you notice food starting to stick more. After each use, simply wipe down the still-warm cooking surface with a thin coat of oil. Then, heat the griddle to medium for 5 to 10 minutes for the oil to re-polymerize. If the seasoning starts to wear off, repeat the initial process to re-season it. You could do this every few months as standard, if you want, too.

BENEFITS OF USING A GAS GRIDDLE

- **Unparalleled Cooking Versatility**

  The expansive, flat cooking surface of a gas griddle lets you cook many different foods on one appliance. You can make burgers, hash browns, pancakes, and steaks all on the same griddle. Plus, with the ability to control the temperature across the entire surface, you can cook multiple items at different heat levels simultaneously. This level of versatility is incredible, letting you streamline your meal prep and save tons of time and effort in the kitchen.

- **Consistent, Even Heating**

  One of the biggest advantages of gas griddles is the even, consistent heat distribution feature across the entire cooking surface. There are no hot or cold spots to worry about, meaning your food will cook evenly and brown beautifully, whether frying a stack of pancakes or making pizza. This even heat is crucial for achieving those perfect, restaurant-quality results at home.

- **Speedy Cooking Times**

  Compared to their electric cousins, gas griddles have a wide speed advantage when heating and sustaining high cooking temperatures. You don't have to wait around for what feels like an eternity for the griddle to preheat fully. Just turn on the burners and you're good to go in much less time. This rapid heating lets you get food on the table faster, a major plus for busy home cooks or commercial kitchens. Waiting for your cooking surface to heat up is the worst, but with a gas griddle, you don't have to waste time twiddling your thumbs.

- **Easy Cleanup**

  Cooking on a griddle will ultimately descend into chaos, but with a gas model, cleanup is surprisingly simple, especially if you've properly seasoned the cooking surface. The flat, smooth griddle top means food, grease, and grime wipe away easily with just a quick wipe-down. Many gas griddles also feature built-in grease management systems, with drip trays or channels to catch all the excess fat and oil. This makes the post-cooking cleanup extremely easy, so you can enjoy your meal in peace without dreading the work that comes after.

- **Durable, Long-lasting Construction**

  A quality gas griddle is built to last, with sturdy stainless steel or cast iron construction that can withstand the demands of frequent, high-heat cooking. These appliances are designed to be durable, standing up to years of heavy use without losing their performance or reliability. With proper care and maintenance, a well-made gas griddle will be a kitchen staple for decades, and you won't have to replace a finicky, less durable model every few years.

Chapter 2:
Breakfast
Bonanza

Mornings are a sacred time, a chance to start the day off right. Unfortunately, for many people, the morning routine might sometimes feel like a race against the clock, but a gas griddle can help simplify the process.

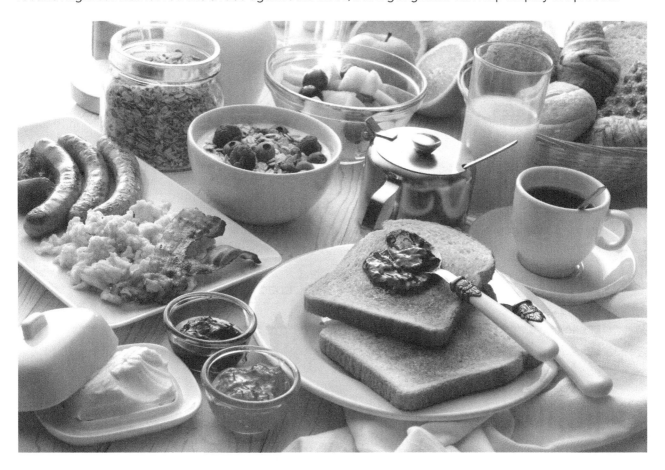

As your alarm threatens your patience, pulling you from a good night's sleep, the to-do list starts scrolling through your mind—shower, get dressed, pack lunches, corral the kids, and, oh yeah, somehow squeeze in a nutritious breakfast all in time for work. It's enough to make your head spin before you've even had that first sip of coffee.

However, mornings become a calmer, more manageable experience with your gas griddle. Rather than frantically darting between the stove, the toaster, and the microwave, simply turn to your griddle, where bacon can sizzle alongside pancakes. And with a few deft flips of the spatula, breakfast comes together in a matter of minutes.

The convenience of a gas griddle extends beyond just the cooking process. Its large, flat cooking area means you can prepare multiple items simultaneously, saving precious time in the morning rush. And with the even heat distribution, you can count on consistent results every single time without worrying about uneven cooking or hot spots. When breakfast is done, cleanup is straightforward. The smooth, flat surface wipes down in a flash, leaving you with one less chore to worry about.

Now that you know what a gas griddle can do for your morning routine, it's time for some of the best morning meal ideas that will have you looking forward to that alarm clock each day.

TIPS FOR MAKING BREAKFAST ON YOUR GRIDDLE

- Shredded potatoes are great but tricky. Squeeze as much moisture as possible out before cooking, then spread them out in a thin, even layer on the hot surface. Avoid messing with them too much so they can brown beautifully.
- Resist the urge to overcrowd your griddle. That'll lead to steaming rather than browning. Cook in small, manageable batches.
- When it's time to flip your pancakes, fritters, or whatever you're cooking, defy the temptation to touch them too soon. Wait until they've nicely browned on the first side before attempting the flip.
- Preheat that griddle properly. You want it nice and hot before you start cooking, so give it a good 5 to 10 minutes before placing anything on top.
- A little bit of oil or butter goes a long way on a griddle. You need just enough to coat the surface lightly. Too much, and you'll end up with a greasy mess, too little, and things will stick.
- Feel free to season your meats, like sausage or bacon, right on the griddle. It tastes even better.

KITCHEN TOOLS NEEDED

- Mixing bowls
- Aluminum foil (Or oven, to keep the food warm)
- Paper towels
- Baking sheet
- Serving plates

BUTTERMILK PANCAKES

Serving: 8
Prep time: 15 mins
Cooking time: 30 mins

There's nothing quite like a stack of light and fluffy buttermilk pancakes to start your day. This recipe is a tried-and-true classic that you will never get tired of. The buttermilk gives the pancakes a nice, tangy flavor, while the vanilla and cinnamon bring warmth and depth. Serve them hot off the griddle with your choice of toppings, like maple syrup, fresh fruit, whipped cream, or even a sprinkle of powdered sugar.

INGREDIENTS:

- 2 cups of all-purpose flour
- 2 teaspoons of baking powder
- 2 tablespoons of white sugar
- 2 cups of buttermilk
- 1 teaspoon of baking soda

- 2 large eggs
- ¼ teaspoon of ground cinnamon
- 4 tablespoons of melted, unsalted butter
- 1 teaspoon of vanilla extract
- ½ teaspoon of salt

DIRECTIONS:

1. Add the salt, baking soda, baking powder, flour, and sugar into a mixing bowl and whisk them.
2. Mix the buttermilk, eggs, melted butter, vanilla, and cinnamon in a different bowl.
3. Pour the buttermilk mixture into the flour mixture and stir until you get a paste, but don't overmix; a few lumps are okay.
4. Heat the gas griddle on medium. Lightly grease the surface with a little butter or nonstick cooking spray.
5. Scoop the batter onto the hot griddle, using about ¼ cup per pancake. Cook for 2 to 3 minutes per side or until cooked through.
6. Serve the pancakes warm, with bacon slices or fruit.

BLUEBERRY PANCAKES

Serving: 4
Prep time: 15 mins
Cooking time: 25 mins

The very thought of blueberry pancakes conjures homesick memories—lazy weekend mornings, the smell of freshly brewed coffee, and the pitter-patter of little feet racing down the stairs. These pancakes somehow transport you to a simpler, more carefree time, and this recipe captures all the familiar and extraordinary flavors of this iconic breakfast.

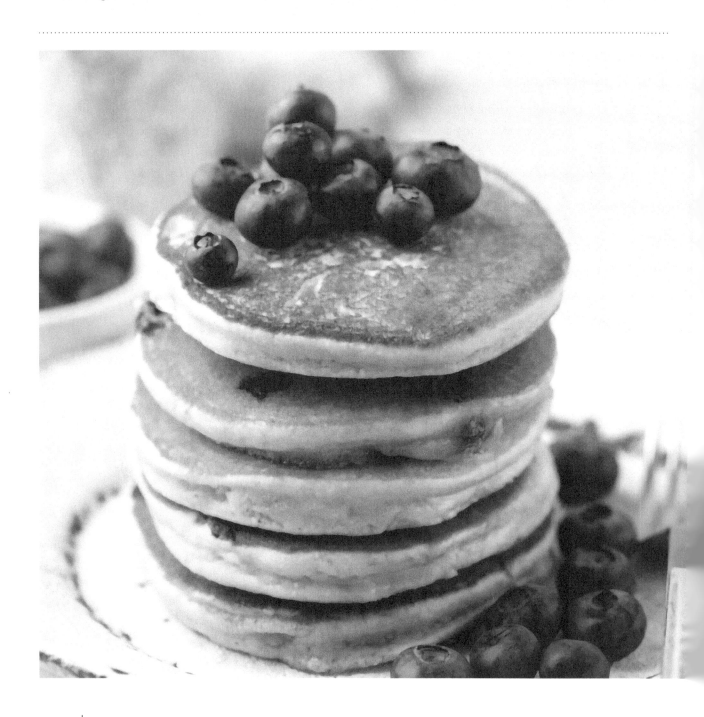

INGREDIENTS:

- 1¼ cups of all-purpose flour
- 3½ teaspoons of baking powder
- 1 tablespoon of white sugar
- ½ teaspoon of salt
- 1¼ cups of milk
- 1 egg
- 3 tablespoons of melted butter
- 1 cup of fresh or frozen blueberries

DIRECTIONS:

1. Mix the flour, baking powder, sugar, and salt in a large bowl.
2. Beat the egg in another bowl. Then, add the milk and melted butter and stir until it is properly mixed.
3. Pour the wet ingredients into the dry ingredients, and use a spoon or spatula to gently fold the mixture until you get a paste. Be careful not to overmix because the result will be tough, rubbery pancakes.
4. Fold in the blueberries, doing your best to see that they are evenly distributed throughout the batter.
5. Preheat your gas griddle on low and grease the surface with butter or a spritz of nonstick cooking spray.
6. Scoop a quarter cup of batter onto the griddle per pancake, spacing them a few inches apart.
7. Cook the pancakes for 2 to 3 minutes, or until bubbles form on the surface and the edges begin to look dry. Flip the pancakes and cook for 1 to 2 minutes or until they look golden brown.
8. Repeat step 7 until you exhaust the batter. Keep the cooked pancakes warm in a low-temperature oven or covered with foil while you finish cooking the rest.
9. Serve the blueberry pancakes warm with whipped cream on top.

FRENCH TOAST

Serving: 8
Prep time: 5 mins
Cooking time: 10 mins

French toast has a long and storied history, with origins that can be traced back centuries to ancient Rome. The basic concept of soaking bread in a custard-type mixture and then cooking it originated as a clever way to use up stale bread. Over time, the dish evolved into a beloved breakfast and comfort food. It's the perfect blend of sweet, eggy, and crunchy.

INGREDIENTS:

- 4 large eggs
- ½ cup of whole milk
- ¼ cup of heavy cream
- 2 tablespoons of white sugar
- 1 teaspoon of ground cinnamon
- ¼ teaspoon of ground nutmeg
- ¼ teaspoon of salt
- 8 slices of day-old or stale bread (such as challah, brioche, or thick-cut Texas toast)
- 2 tablespoons of unsalted butter.

DIRECTIONS:

1. Mix the eggs, milk, heavy cream, sugar, cinnamon, nutmeg, and salt in a large, shallow bowl.
2. Preheat your gas griddle on medium heat and grease the surface with a thin layer of butter.
3. One at a time, dip the bread slices into the egg mix and let them soak up the custard on both sides. Gently shake off any excess before placing the coated bread slices onto the hot griddle.
4. Cook the French toast for 2 to 3 minutes per side until golden and crispy. You may need to work in batches, depending on the size of your griddle.
5. Flip the French toast slices carefully using a spatula, mindful not to tear the delicate, custard-soaked bread.
6. Once both sides are evenly cooked, transfer the toast to a warm oven (around 200°F) to keep it crisp and toasty while cooking the remaining slices.
7. Serve the French toast hot with your favorite toppings. Maple syrup, powdered sugar, fresh fruit, or a dollop of whipped cream are popular choices.

HAM AND SWISS GRIDDLE MELTS

Serving: 4
Prep time: 10 mins
Cooking time: 20 mins

Ham and Swiss griddle melts are made by sandwiching slices of deli-style ham and Swiss cheese between two pieces of thick-cut sourdough or artisan bread. The sandwiches are then cooked to create a crispy, golden brown exterior while the cheese gets melted and gooey inside.

INGREDIENTS:

- 8 slices of thick-cut sourdough or artisan bread
- 8 slices of Swiss cheese
- 8 thin slices of deli-style ham
- 4 tablespoons of softened, unsalted butter

DIRECTIONS:

1. Preheat your gas griddle on medium heat.
2. Spread a very thin layer of butter on 1 side of each slice of bread. This will be the outside of your sandwiches.
3. Place 4 slices of bread, butter-side down, on the hot griddle. Top each slice with 2 slices of Swiss cheese and 2 slices of ham.
4. Place the remaining 4 slices of bread, butter-side up, on top of the cheese and ham to form the sandwiches.
5. Cook the griddle melts for 3 to 4 minutes per side or until the bread is brown and the cheese is melted and bubbly. You may need to press down gently on the sandwiches with a spatula to help the cheese melt.
6. Flip the sandwiches carefully, using a spatula to support the bottom slice of bread, and cook for 3 to 4 minutes on the other side until both sides are crispy and the cheese is fully melted.
7. Remove the griddle melts from the heat and let them cool for a minute or two before serving.
8. Slice the sandwiches in half diagonally, if you like, and serve them warm with a side of mustard, pickle slices, or a salad.

APPLE CINNAMON OATMEAL CAKES

Serving: 2
Prep time: 10 mins
Cooking time: 15 mins

These oatmeal cakes are perfect for busy mornings when you want something more substantial than a typical muffin or granola bar. Top them with a dollop of yogurt, some maple syrup, or a sprinkle of chopped nuts.

INGREDIENTS:

- 1 cup of old-fashioned oats
- 1 cup of all-purpose flour
- 2 teaspoons of baking powder
- 1 teaspoon of ground cinnamon
- ¼ teaspoon of salt
- 1 cup of milk
- 1 large egg

- 2 tablespoons of melted unsalted butter
- 2 tablespoons of brown sugar
- 1 teaspoon of vanilla extract
- 1 cup of peeled and diced apple (1 medium-sized apple)
- Butter or nonstick cooking spray

DIRECTIONS:

1. Mix the dry ingredients in a bowl: the oats, flour, baking powder, cinnamon, and salt.
2. Pour the milk, egg, melted butter, brown sugar, and vanilla into a separate bowl. Mix thoroughly.
3. Pour the wet ingredients into the dry ingredients and stir until you get a fairly consistent paste. Gently fold in the diced apple.
4. Preheat your gas griddle on medium heat. Grease the surface with a bit of butter or nonstick cooking spray.
5. Scoop the batter onto the hot griddle, leaving a few inches between each cake.
6. Cook the cakes for 2 to 3 minutes or until you see bubbles on the surface and the edges look set.
7. Flip the cakes and cook for 1 to 2 more minutes until they look golden brown on both sides.
8. Repeat with the remaining batter. Cover the cooked cakes with foil while you finish cooking the rest.
9. Serve your apple cinnamon oatmeal cakes warm with fresh apple slices on top.

VEGGIE FRITTATA

Serving: 2
Prep time: 10 mins
Cooking time: 10 mins

This crustless quiche or baked egg dish is the supreme breakfast option when you want something nutritious but not too heavy.

INGREDIENTS:

- 4 large eggs
- 2 tablespoon of unsweetened almond milk (or regular milk)
- A pinch of salt
- A pinch of black pepper
- 2 teaspoon of olive oil

- 4 tablespoons of diced bell pepper
- 4 tablespoons of sliced mushrooms
- 2 tablespoon of diced onion
- 4 tablespoons of shredded cheddar cheese
- 2 teaspoon of chopped fresh parsley (optional)

DIRECTIONS:

1. Preheat your gas griddle on medium heat.
2. In a small bowl, beat the eggs, almond milk, salt, and pepper.
3. Add the olive oil to the hot griddle and brush to coat the surface. This will help your frittata release easily when it's time to flip.
4. Pour the egg mixture onto the griddle, making a big round frittata. You might need a ring or mold to keep the egg mixture together.
5. Top the frittata with the diced bell pepper, mushrooms, and onion.
6. Cook the frittata for 2 to 3 minutes, until the edges are set and the bottom is lightly browned.
7. Carefully flip the frittata and cook for 1 to 2 minutes until the center is cooked through.
8. Top the frittata with the shredded cheddar cheese.
9. Cover the griddle with a lid or baking sheet and cook for 1 or 2 minutes more until the cheese is melted.
10. Transfer the veggie frittata to a plate and garnish with chopped fresh parsley, if you like.
11. Serve with fresh berries on the side.

AVOCADO TOAST

Serving: 2
Prep time: 8 mins
Cooking time: 15 mins

Want something quick and simple? This recipe has you covered. It's the ultimate guilt-free indulgence—healthy but still utterly satisfying. The best part is you can dress it up or down however you like.

INGREDIENTS:

- 2 slices of whole-grain bread
- 1 ripe avocado, pitted and mashed
- 1 tablespoon of olive oil
- ¼ teaspoon of salt
- A pinch of black pepper

- 1 tablespoon of crumbled feta cheese (optional)
- 1 teaspoon of everything bagel seasoning (optional)

DIRECTIONS:

1. Preheat your griddle on medium heat.
2. Mash the avocado in a small bowl, then add the olive oil, salt, and pepper. Mix everything until you reach a smooth consistency.
3. Place the bread slices directly on the hot griddle and toast for 2 to 3 minutes per side until crispy and golden brown.
4. Remove the toasted bread from the griddle and immediately top each slice with the mashed avocado paste.
5. If using, sprinkle the crumbled feta cheese and everything bagel seasoning over the avocado toasts.
6. Serve the avocado toast warm with onion rings or scrambled eggs.

BREAKFAST POTATO HASH

Serving: 2
Prep time: 10 mins
Cooking time: 20 mins

The basic premise of a breakfast potato hash is cubed or shredded potatoes that are sautéed with other ingredients, usually onions, peppers, and different seasonings. Want to keep it simple? Just toss the potatoes with some spices and call it a day. Feeling fancy? Throw in all the fixings—cheese, herbs, even a runny egg on top.

INGREDIENTS:

- 2 medium russet potatoes, peeled and diced into ½-inch cubes (about 2 cups)
- 2 tablespoons of olive oil
- ½ lb. of breakfast sausage, casings removed and crumbled
- ½ cup of diced bell pepper
- ¼ cup of diced onion
- 1 teaspoon of garlic powder

- 1 teaspoon of smoked paprika
- ½ teaspoon of salt
- ¼ teaspoon of black pepper
- 2 large eggs, cooked to preferred doneness (optional)
- 2 tablespoons of chopped fresh parsley (optional)

DIRECTIONS:

1. Preheat your griddle on medium-high heat.
2. Pour the diced potatoes onto the hot griddle and leave it to cook. Stir every now and then for 8 to 10 minutes until the potatoes are starting to brown and look crispy on the outside.
3. Push the potatoes to one side of the griddle, then add the crumbled breakfast sausage to the empty space. Cook the sausage for 3 to 4 minutes, breaking it up with a spatula as it cooks until it is browned and cooked through.
4. Add the diced bell pepper and onion to the griddle. Cook for 2 to 3 minutes, stirring everything together, until the vegetables are softened.
5. Stir in the garlic powder, smoked paprika, salt, and black pepper. Cook for 1 more minute to toast the spices.
6. Remove the hash from the griddle and top each serving with a fried or scrambled egg and a sprinkle of fresh, chopped parsley.

BREAKFAST BISCUITS WITH JAM

Serving: 8
Prep time: 12 mins
Cooking time: 10 mins

There's something undeniably nostalgic and homey about this combination. It's the kind of simple, old-fashioned breakfast that feels comforting and familiar, like something your grandma used to make. Despite its simplicity, it's a breakfast that makes you feel good.

INGREDIENTS:

- 2 cups of all-purpose flour
- 2 teaspoons of baking powder
- ½ teaspoon of salt
- 5 tablespoons of cold, cubed, unsalted butter
- ¾ cup of cold buttermilk
- ¼ cup of your favorite jam or preserves

DIRECTIONS:

1. Preheat your griddle on medium-high heat.
2. Mix the flour, baking powder, and salt in a bowl.
3. Throw in the cold cubed butter and use your fingertips to quickly work it into the dry ingredients until the mixture resembles coarse crumbs with a few pea-sized pieces of butter remaining.
4. Add the chilled buttermilk and whisk just long enough to form a shaggy dough. Mixing after this is not advised.
5. After transferring the dough to a lightly floured surface, gently knead it for 2 to 3 minutes to bring it together.
6. Pat the dough into a ¾-inch-thick round. Use a 2-inch biscuit cutter to cut out 8 biscuits, pressing straight down without twisting.
7. Carefully transfer the biscuits to the preheated griddle, leaving just enough space between them.
8. Let the biscuits cook for 3 to 4 minutes per side or until they brown on both sides.
9. Take them off the griddle and let them cool for 5 minutes.
10. Split the biscuits in half, spread each side with your favorite jam, and serve alongside chocolate milk.

Chapter 3:
Sandwiches and Quesadillas

You know what they say—the best things in life come in handheld packages. Sandwiches and quesadillas may play by different rules, but their sheer convenience is hard to beat. Easily assembled and equally easy to eat on the go, they are the best solution for busy schedules, road trips, or moments when you need a quick yet filling meal. With a gas griddle, the trick is patience and a watchful eye. The dry, even heat will deliver a flawlessly toasted exterior and a warm, melty interior every time. This may be easy, but it's anything but basic.

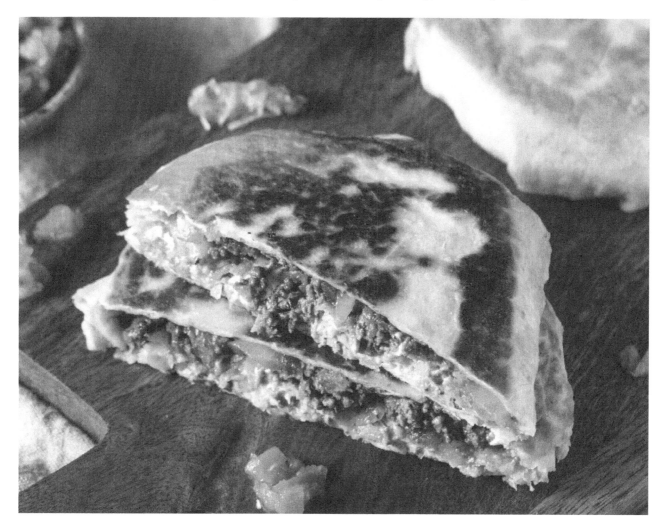

Tips for Making Sandwiches and Quesadillas on a Gas Griddle

- When assembling your sandwich fillings, layer heavier items like cheese and meats in the center, with vegetables and condiments on the outer edges.
- For quesadillas, use freshly grated cheese or small cheese slices so they melt evenly throughout.
- Brush the top tortilla with a little oil or melted butter before flipping the quesadilla. This guarantees even browning.
- Try brushing the bread or tortillas with garlic butter, pesto, or a thin layer of your favorite spread for extra flavor.
- For sandwiches, spread a thin layer of mayonnaise or butter on the outside of the bread before grilling. This creates an amazing, crispy exterior.

- Let your sandwiches or quesadillas rest for a minute or two after cooking. This gives the fillings a chance to settle.
- Experiment with different flavor combinations. You'd be surprised what works well grilled together.

KITCHEN TOOLS NEEDED

- Mixing bowls
- Cutting board
- Sandwich press
- Food processor
- Serving plates

CHICKEN PESTO PANINI

Serving: 2
Prep time: 10 mins
Cooking time: 20 mins

A panini is an Italian-style grilled sandwich made by pressing the ingredients between two pieces of bread and grilling them on a heated surface until the bread is toasted and the fillings are hot and melted. This chicken pesto panini features tender chicken, basil pesto, and mozzarella cheese, all sandwiched between two slices of crusty bread.

INGREDIENTS:

- 8 ounces of boneless, skinless chicken breast
- ½ teaspoon of salt
- A pinch of black pepper
- 3 teaspoons of olive oil

- 4 slices of sourdough or ciabatta bread
- 2 tablespoons of basil pesto
- 4 ounces of fresh mozzarella cheese, sliced

DIRECTIONS:

1. Season the chicken breast with salt and pepper.
2. Heat your griddle on medium-high. Drizzle the olive oil over the surface and cook the chicken for 5 to 6 minutes per side until cooked through. Transfer the chicken to a cutting board and let it rest for 5 minutes, then slice or shred it.
3. Spread 1 tablespoon of pesto on 1 slice of bread. Top with the sliced chicken and mozzarella cheese slices.
4. Place the remaining slice of bread on top to make a sandwich.
5. Preheat your gas griddle to medium-high again.
6. Place the panini on the hot griddle. Use a sandwich press to press down on the sandwich as it cooks. Cook for 3 to 4 minutes per side or until the bread is toasted and the cheese has melted.
7. Remove the panini from the griddle and let it rest for 2 minutes before serving with zucchini fries (Pg. 142).

CUBANO

Serving: 4
Prep time: 5 mins
Cooking time: 25 mins

The Cubano, or Cuban sandwich, is a pressed and grilled sandwich that originated in Cuba and became popular in Cuban-American communities, especially in Florida. It has two slices of soft, slightly sweet Cuban bread between Swiss cheese, several pieces of thinly sliced roast pork, pickles, ham, and mustard.

INGREDIENTS:

- 8 ounces of sliced roast pork
- 4 ounces of sliced ham
- 4 ounces of thinly sliced Swiss cheese
- 8 slices of dill pickle chips
- 2 tablespoons of yellow mustard
- 4 soft Cuban or French bread rolls, split lengthwise

DIRECTIONS:

1. Heat your griddle on medium.
2. Layer the bottom half of each bread roll with the roast pork, ham, Swiss cheese, and pickles. Spread the mustard on the top half of the rolls.
3. Close the sandwiches and place them on the hot griddle. Use a heavy pan or sandwich press to press down on the sandwiches as they cook.
4. Grill the sandwiches for 3 to 4 minutes on each side until the cheese is melted and the bread looks toasted.
5. Remove the Cubanos from the griddle and let them rest for 2 minutes before serving. They go really well with potato chips.

WALLEYE SANDWICH

Serving: 2
Prep time: 12 mins
Cooking time: 20 mins

The main ingredient here is walleye, and it's kind of a big deal, especially if you're into fishing or good seafood. Walleye are freshwater fish that are native to lakes and rivers across North America, and they're known for their flaky white meat that tastes absolutely amazing. The fish puts up a good fight on the line, so they are really tough to catch, but when you do reel one in and go the extra mile to put it in a sandwich, that's where things get really good.

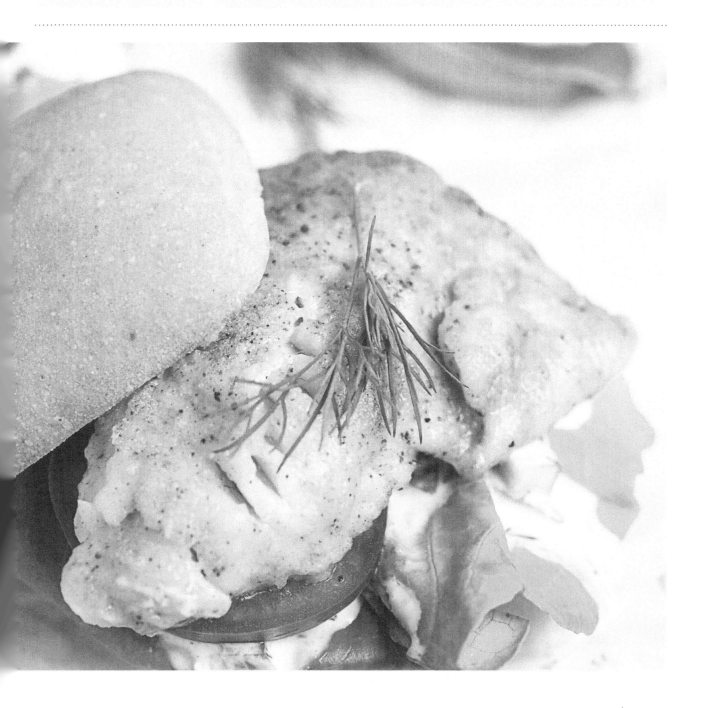

INGREDIENTS:

- 2 walleye filets
- ½ cup of all-purpose flour
- 2 beaten eggs
- 1 cup of panko breadcrumbs
- 1 teaspoon of salt
- ½ teaspoon of black pepper

- 2 tablespoons of olive oil
- 2 soft hamburger buns, split
- 2 tablespoons of tartar sauce
- 2 lettuce leaves
- 2 tomato slices

DIRECTIONS:

1. Pat the walleye filets dry with paper towels. Season both sides with salt and pepper.
2. Set up a breading station with the flour in one bowl, the beaten eggs in another, and the panko breadcrumbs in a third bowl.
3. Dredge the walleye filets in the flour, dip them in the egg, and then coat them with the panko breadcrumbs, pressing to make them stick.
4. Heat your gas griddle on medium-high and pour the olive oil on the surface.
5. Carefully place the breaded walleye filets on the hot griddle, working in batches if necessary. Cook for 3 to 4 minutes per side or until they are golden brown and cooked through.
6. Toast the buns on the griddle for 1 to 2 minutes until they look light brown.
7. To assemble the sandwiches, spread 1 tablespoon of tartar sauce on the bottom bun. Top with a walleye filet, a lettuce leaf, and a tomato slice. Close with the top bun and serve with roasted asparagus.

CHICKEN CAPRESE SANDWICH

Serving: 2
Prep time: 10 mins
Cooking time: 25 mins

Have you ever bitten into a sandwich that takes you straight to the sun-drenched Italian countryside? That's exactly what this chicken caprese sandwich will do.

INGREDIENTS:

- 2 boneless, skinless chicken breasts
- 1 teaspoon of olive oil
- 1 teaspoon of dried Italian seasoning
- ½ teaspoon of salt
- ¼ teaspoon of black pepper

- 2 ciabatta or sandwich rolls, split in half
- 4 ounces of fresh mozzarella cheese, sliced
- 1 sliced tomato
- 6 fresh basil leaves

DIRECTIONS:

1. Heat your gas griddle on medium-high.
2. Grab the chicken breasts and rub them with the olive oil, Italian seasoning, salt, and pepper. You want every inch of that chicken coated in the seasonings.
3. Carefully place the seasoned chicken on the hot griddle. Let them cook for 5 to 7 minutes per side until they're cooked through and reach 165°F on a thermometer. Once done, transfer them to a cutting board and let them rest for 5 minutes before slicing or shredding.
4. While the chicken rests, place the ciabatta or sandwich rolls cut-side down on the griddle for 1 to 2 minutes until they're golden and crisp.
5. Layer the bottom half of each roll with some of the seasoned chicken. Top it off with slices of fresh mozzarella, tomato, and a few basil leaves.
6. Put the sandwiches back on the griddle and use a sandwich press to press them down as they cook for another 2 to 3 minutes per side. This will melt the cheese and crisp the bread even further.
7. Remove the sandwiches from the griddle and serve them hot.

MONTE CRISTO

Serving: 2
Prep time: 7 mins
Cooking time: 16 mins

The Monte Cristo sandwich is the stuff that breakfast dreams are made of. This decadent creation takes the grilled cheese sandwich to the next level, fusing sweet and savory in this interplay of ham, turkey, cheese, and custard-soaked bread.

INGREDIENTS:

- 4 slices of white bread
- 2 eggs
- ¼ cup of milk
- 1 tablespoon of granulated sugar
- ¼ teaspoon of ground cinnamon

- 2 ounces of sliced deli ham
- 2 ounces of sliced deli turkey
- 4 slices of Swiss cheese
- Powdered sugar for dusting (optional)

DIRECTIONS:

1. Beat the eggs, milk, granulated sugar, and cinnamon in a bowl.
2. Heat your griddle on medium.
3. Dip 2 slices of bread into the egg mixture, coating both sides.
4. Place the slices of egg-coated bread on the hot griddle and cook them on both sides for 2 minutes each. Top each slice with 1 ounce of ham, 1 ounce of turkey, and 2 slices of Swiss cheese.
5. Cover the sandwiches with the remaining 2 slices of bread.
6. Cook the Monte Cristo sandwiches for 3 to 4 minutes per side until the bread is golden brown and the cheese is melted.
7. Transfer the hot sandwiches to a cutting board. Slice each sandwich diagonally in half.
8. Serve the Monte Cristo sandwiches warm, dusted with powdered sugar.

REUBEN SANDWICH

Serving: 2
Prep time: 10 mins
Cooking time: 16 mins

The origins of the Reuben sandwich are somewhat disputed, but it's generally believed to have been created in the early 20th century. The most widely accepted story is that it was invented in 1914 by a Jewish-American grocer named Reuben Kulakofsky in Omaha, Nebraska. He created the sandwich for a poker game he hosted, and it didn't waste any time becoming a popular menu item at the Blackstone Hotel, where the games took place and across the world.

INGREDIENTS:

- 4 slices of rye bread
- 2 tablespoons of butter, softened
- 4 ounces of thinly sliced corned beef
- 1 cup of sauerkraut, drained and patted dry
- 4 slices of Swiss cheese
- ½ cup of Thousand Island dressing

DIRECTIONS:

1. Heat your griddle on medium.
2. Spread the softened butter evenly on one side of each slice of rye bread.
3. Place 2 slices of the bread, butter-side down, on the hot griddle.
4. Layer each bread slice with 2 ounces of corned beef, ¼ cup of sauerkraut, 2 slices of Swiss cheese, and 2 tablespoons of Thousand Island dressing.
5. Top each sandwich with the remaining 2 slices of bread, butter-side up.
6. Cook the Reuben sandwiches for 3 to 4 minutes per side or until the bread is perfectly toasted and the cheese has melted.
7. Transfer the hot Reuben sandwiches to a cutting board and use a sharp knife to diagonally slice each sandwich in half.
8. Serve the Reuben sandwiches warm, with extra Thousand Island dressing for dipping if you like.

BRISKET AND CARAMELIZED ONION QUESADILLA

Serving: 4
Prep time: 5 mins
Cooking time: 35 mins

This recipe is a fusion of Tex-Mex and slow-cooked comfort food flavors. While the exact origins are a bit vague, this quesadilla reflects the creative and delicious ways that Tex-Mex chefs and home cooks have put their own spin on classic Mexican dishes over the decades. The result is a boldly flavored quesadilla with layers of meat, sweet onions, and melted cheese, all wrapped in a golden shell.

INGREDIENTS:

- 4 ounces of cooked, shredded beef brisket (Pg. 47)
- 1 large, thinly sliced yellow onion
- 1 tablespoon of butter
- 1 tablespoon of brown sugar
- A pinch of salt
- 2 large flour tortillas
- ½ cup of shredded cheddar cheese
- ½ cup of shredded mozzarella cheese

DIRECTIONS:

1. On your griddle over medium-low heat, melt the butter. Add the sliced onion and stir now and then for 25 to 30 minutes until the onion is very soft and caramelized. Stir in the brown sugar and salt. Scoop the caramelized onion off the griddle and set it aside.
2. Place 1 of the flour tortillas on the hot griddle. Divide the shredded brisket, caramelized onion, cheddar cheese, and mozzarella cheese evenly on the tortilla, leaving a ½ inch border.
3. Top with the remaining flour tortilla.
4. Cook the quesadilla for 2 to 3 minutes per side, using a spatula to press down on it, until the tortilla is golden brown and the cheese has melted.
5. Remove the quesadilla from the griddle and cut it into 4 triangular wedges.

MANGO AND HABANERO CHICKEN QUESADILLA

Serving: 4
Prep time: 10 mins
Cooking time: 30 mins

This quesadilla is very easy to make at home. You only need a few simple ingredients: chicken, mango, cheese, tortillas, and a couple of spices. Throw it all together, give it a good sear in your griddle and you are promised a party in your mouth.

INGREDIENTS:

- 1 lb. of boneless, skinless chicken breasts
- 2 teaspoons of chili powder
- 1 teaspoon of ground cumin
- ½ teaspoon of garlic powder
- ¼ teaspoon of salt
- ¼ teaspoon of black pepper
- 1 ripe mango, peeled and diced

- 1 habanero pepper, seeded and finely chopped
- 8 (8-inch) flour tortillas
- 2 cups of shredded Monterey Jack cheese
- Sour cream, cilantro, and lime wedges for serving

DIRECTIONS:

1. Season the chicken breasts on both sides with chili powder, cumin, garlic powder, salt, and pepper.
2. Preheat your griddle on medium-high heat. Cook the seasoned chicken for 5 to 7 minutes per side or until cooked through. Leave the chicken to rest for 5 minutes, then shred or dice it.
3. Mix the shredded chicken, diced mango, and chopped habanero in a bowl. Mix them well.
4. Place 4 of the flour tortillas on the hot griddle. Divide the chicken-mango mixture evenly among the tortillas, spreading it out to the edges. Sprinkle ½ cup of the shredded Monterey Jack cheese over each one.
5. Top each quesadilla with the remaining 4 tortillas.
6. Cook the quesadillas for 2 to 3 minutes per side. Use a spatula to flatten it gently. Cook until the tortillas are golden brown and the cheese has melted.
7. Remove the quesadillas from the griddle and cut each one into 4 triangular wedges.
8. Serve immediately with sour cream, chopped cilantro, and lime wedges on the side.

SHREDDED BEEF AND CHIMICHURRI QUESADILLA

Serving: 4
Prep time: 10 mins
Cooking time: 12 mins

If the essence of chimichurri sauce could be explained in a single word, it'd probably be "bright." When spooned over the flavored shredded beef, the chimichurri's bright, assertive character cuts straight through the fattiness of the meat. This contrast is what makes this quesadilla so craveable.

INGREDIENTS:

- 4 ounces of cooked, shredded chuck roast or brisket (Pgs. 47 and 48 respectively)
- ¼ cup of loosely packed fresh parsley leaves
- 2 tablespoons of olive oil
- 1 minced garlic clove
- 1 teaspoon of red wine vinegar
- A pinch or more of red pepper flakes
- A pinch of salt
- 2 (8-inch) flour tortillas
- ½ cup shredded Oaxaca or Monterey Jack cheese

DIRECTIONS:

1. Put the parsley, olive oil, garlic, red wine vinegar, oregano, red pepper flakes, and salt into a food processor. Pulse until a coarse chimichurri sauce forms. Set it aside.
2. Preheat your griddle on medium heat.
3. Place 1 of the flour tortillas on the hot griddle. Spread the shredded beef evenly over the tortilla, then spoon 2 to 3 tablespoons of the chimichurri sauce over the beef. Sprinkle half a cup of the shredded cheese over the top.
4. Top with the remaining flour tortilla.
5. Cook the quesadilla for 2 to 3 minutes per side and use a spatula to press down gently. The quesadilla is fully cooked when the tortilla is brown and the cheese is melted.
6. Take the quesadilla off the griddle and cut it into 4 triangular wedges.
7. Serve warm with extra chimichurri sauce, sour cream, chopped cilantro, and lime wedges on the side.

PHILLY CHEESESTEAK QUESADILLA

Serving: 2
Prep time: 7 mins
Cooking time: 20 mins

If you happen to have leftover sliced steak or roast beef in the fridge, you're already halfway through this super easy recipe. Simply chop it up and use it as the base for the quesadilla filling.

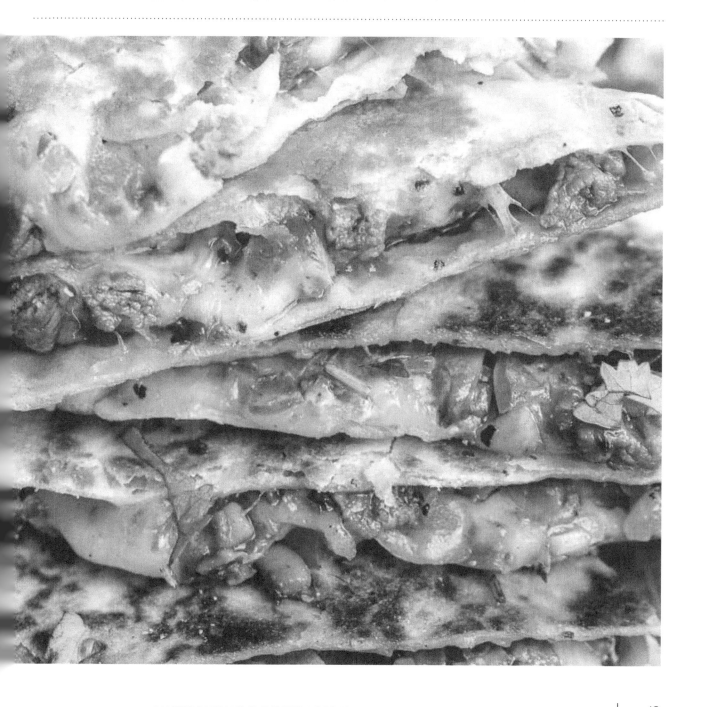

INGREDIENTS:

- 4 ounces of thinly sliced ribeye or sirloin steak
- ½ onion, thinly sliced
- ½ green bell pepper, thinly sliced
- 1 tablespoon of vegetable oil
- ½ teaspoon of garlic powder
- ½ teaspoon of dried oregano
- ¼ teaspoon of salt
- A pinch of black pepper
- 2 (8-inch) flour tortillas
- 4 ounces of provolone cheese, sliced
- Sour cream, pickled peppers, and parsley for serving

DIRECTIONS:

1. Heat your griddle on medium-high and add the vegetable oil. Throw in the sliced steak, onions, and bell peppers. Cook for 5 to 7 minutes, stirring now and then, until the vegetables are soft and the steak is cooked through.
2. Season that mixture with the garlic powder, oregano, salt, and pepper. Give it a good stir to distribute the seasonings evenly.
3. Lay one of the tortillas down on the hot griddle. Scoop half of the steak and veggie mixture onto the tortilla, spreading it out to the edges. Top that with 2 ounces of the provolone cheese slices.
4. To complete your quesadilla, place the other tortilla on top. Allow it to cook on each side for 2 to 3 minutes, using a spatula to gently press down so the cheese melts.
5. Once the tortilla is golden brown and the cheese is melted, remove your quesadilla from the griddle and cut it into 4 triangles.
6. Serve them hot with a dollop of sour cream, some pickled peppers, and a sprinkle of fresh parsley.

SOUTHWESTERN BLACK BEAN QUESADILLA (VEGAN)

Serving: 2
Prep time: 10 mins
Cooking time: 12 mins

If you're looking for something wholesome and easy to prepare, look no further than these Southwestern black bean quesadillas. You don't even have to cook the filling; just throw all the ingredients into a bowl, and you're ready to assemble.

INGREDIENTS:

- 1 can of black beans, rinsed and drained
- ½ onion, diced
- ½ red bell pepper, diced
- 1 tablespoon of olive oil
- 1 teaspoon of ground cumin
- 1 teaspoon of chili powder

- ¼ teaspoon of garlic powder
- ¼ teaspoon of salt
- 2 (8-inch) flour tortillas
- 1 cup of shredded Vegan cheese
- Vegan Sour cream, lime wedges, and Pico de Gallo for serving

DIRECTIONS:

1. Pour the black beans, onion, garlic, cumin, chili powder, and cayenne into a bowl. Season with a pinch of salt and pepper, and stir.
2. Preheat your gas griddle on medium heat.
3. Place one tortilla on the hot griddle. Sprinkle a quarter cup of the shredded cheese onto half of the tortilla. Top with a couple of spoonfuls of the black bean mixture. Fold the other half of the tortilla over the filling.
4. Cook for 2 to 3 minutes per side until the tortilla is light brown and the cheese has melted.
5. Repeat with the remaining tortillas and fillings.
6. Slice each quesadilla in half and serve hot with sides like salsa, sour cream, or guacamole.

SPINACH AND FETA QUESADILLA (VEGETARIAN)

Serving: 2
Prep time: 5 mins
Cooking time: 10 mins

People have been sneaking spinach into their smoothies for years, so why not apply that same concept to the quesadilla? Now, you can eat more greens without sacrificing flavor or satisfaction.

INGREDIENTS:

- 2 medium flour tortilla
- 3 cups of fresh spinach leaves
- 2 tablespoon of olive oil
- 4 tablespoons of crumbled feta cheese
- ½ cup of shredded mozzarella cheese

DIRECTIONS:

1. Preheat your gas griddle on medium heat.
2. Place the tortilla on the hot griddle. Let it warm for 30 to 60 seconds.
3. Toss the fresh spinach leaves with olive oil in a small bowl. You need the leaves coated just barely.
4. Arrange the oiled spinach leaves over half of the tortilla on the griddle. Sprinkle the crumbled feta cheese and shredded mozzarella cheese evenly over the spinach.
5. Fold the empty half of the tortilla over the filled half to create a half-moon shape.
6. Cook the quesadilla for 2 to 3 minutes per side until the tortilla is golden brown and the cheeses are melted.
7. Remove the quesadilla from the griddle and let it cool for a minute or two.
8. Slice the quesadilla in half and serve hot, with sweet potato fries if you have some.

BEEF BRISKET

Serving: 4
Prep time: 5 mins
Cooking time: 3 hrs 10 mins

INGREDIENTS:

- 1 pound of beef brisket
- 1 teaspoon of sweet paprika
- 1 tablespoon of sugar
- ¼ teaspoon of cayenne pepper

- ½ teaspoon of onion powder
- 2 teaspoons of salt
- ½ teaspoon of black pepper

DIRECTIONS:

1. Pour the sugar, salt, paprika, onion powder, black pepper, and cayenne pepper into a bowl and mix.
2. Take the brisket and rub the seasoning mix all over the outside of it. Let that sit on the counter for 30 minutes to absorb the flavors.
3. Turn on only one section of your griddle and set it to medium-low heat.
4. Place the seasoned brisket directly on the surface. Let it cook for 5 minutes, then flip it over and cook for 5 more minutes.
5. After searing the brisket on both sides, move it to the other side of the griddle that isn't heated, but the heated portion should remain as it is.
6. Close the lid on your griddle and let the brisket cook on indirect heat for 2 to 3 hours, flipping it over every 30 minutes or so. The brisket is done when it's fork-tender.
7. In the last 30 minutes of cooking, flip the brisket over so the fatty side is facing down on the griddle. Then, use a basting brush to go over the top with your favorite barbecue sauce.
8. Remove the fully cooked brisket from the griddle and let it rest on a cutting board for 10 minutes before slicing it into strips.

CHUCK ROAST

Serving: 4
Prep time: 12 hrs 45 mins
Cooking time: 1 hrs

INGREDIENTS:

- ¼ cup balsamic vinegar
- 2 tablespoons extra-virgin olive oil
- 3 cloves garlic, grated or minced
- 1 teaspoon kosher salt
- 1 teaspoon freshly ground black pepper
- 1 (1 pound) chuck roast
- Flaky sea salt

DIRECTIONS:

1. Mix the balsamic vinegar, olive oil, garlic, kosher salt, and black pepper in a large bowl. Place the chuck roast in the bowl and turn it to coat the meat in the marinade.

2. Cover the bowl and refrigerate for at least 12 hours, turning it over halfway through.

3. Take the chuck roast out of the fridge and let it sit at room temperature for 30 minutes.

4. Preheat your griddle on medium-high heat.

5. Place the marinated chuck roast on the griddle surface. Let it cook for 5 minutes, flip it, and cook for another 5 minutes.

6. Keep turning the roast every 5 minutes, until a thermometer inserted into the thickest part reads 135°F for rare, 140°F for medium-rare, or 145°F for medium.

7. Transfer it to a cutting board and cover it loosely with foil. Let the meat rest for 10 minutes.

8. After the resting period, use a sharp knife to thinly slice the chuck roast against the grain.

9. Sprinkle the slices with a little flaky sea salt before serving or using.

SIRLOIN STEAK

Serving: 4
Prep time: 10 mins
Cooking time: 10 mins

INGREDIENTS:

- ¾ pound of Sirloin steak
- 1 tablespoon of olive oil
- ¼ teaspoon of minced garlic
- 2 tablespoons of softened butter
- ½ tablespoon minced fresh herbs like parsley, chives, or thyme
- Salt and pepper for seasoning

DIRECTIONS:

1. Pat your sirloin dry with a paper towel.
2. Season it with salt and pepper on both sides.
3. Preheat your griddle on medium-high heat and pour olive oil on the surface.
4. Place your sirloin on the griddle and cook each side for 4 to 5 minutes or until it is browned.
5. Stick a thermometer in the steak to check its internal temperature. You'll be cooking it to medium doneness, which is 145°F.
6. While the steak is cooking, get a small bowl and mix the softened butter, minced garlic, and fresh herbs. Season that with a pinch of salt and pepper.
7. If the steak is ready, transfer it to a cutting board and allow it to rest for 5 minutes.
8. Slice it into strips, then top each strip with a scoop of garlic-herb butter.

Chapter 4:
Acts of
Kindness

Engaging in acts of kindness without expecting anything in return has been shown to boost happiness and life satisfaction.

I invite you to embrace that wonderful feeling during your reading today.

It only takes a few moments to answer a simple question:

Would you be willing to make a positive impact in the life of a stranger—without spending any money or seeking recognition?

If so, I have a small favor to ask.

If you've enjoyed your reading experience today, please take a moment to leave an honest review of this book. It will only take about 30 seconds to share your thoughts with others.

Your review can help someone else discover the same inspiration and knowledge you've found.

If you're familiar with leaving reviews for Kindle or e-reader books, it's easy:

For Kindle or e-reader users, simply scroll to the last page and swipe up to leave your review.

For those with a paperback or other physical formats, you can find the book page on Amazon (or wherever you purchased it) and leave your review there.

Your voice can make a difference. Thank you for your support!

Chapter 5:
Burgers

Someone once said, "The only way to eat a burger is with both hands," and they were absolutely right. It is not meant to be delicately nibbled with a fork and knife. Burgers demand to be held, squeezed, and bitten into.

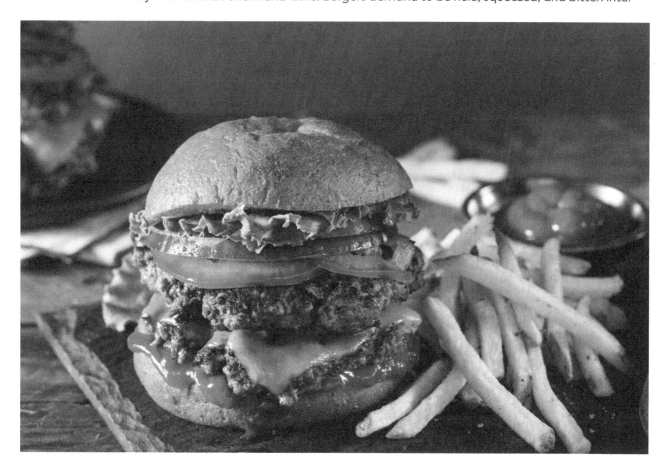

There's an almost primal satisfaction in wrapping your hands around a burger and taking a big, juicy bite. The bun soaks up the burger juices, your fingers get a bit greasy, and the sauce may dribble down your chin. It's messy, but that's the whole point. Anything less would be an incomplete burger experience.

Everyone who loves burgers has the Germans to thank for that. The modern hamburger, as you know it, is rooted in the Hamburg steak, a meal enjoyed by German immigrants in the United States back in the late 19th century. These early Hamburg steaks were essentially ground beef patties, often served between two slices of bread. As the dish blew up, bakers started creating specialized buns to hold the patties, and the hamburger was born.

Thanks to its even heat distribution and precise temperature control, the gas griddle is the perfect tool for making the perfect burger. The flat, evenly heated surface lets you cook the patties to a beautiful, caramelized sear on the outside while ensuring the inside is cooked just right, no matter how you like it. Plus, the big, flat surface can hold multiple patties simultaneously, which is great when feeding a crowd. Never again will you juggle burgers on a tiny grill or have them fall through the cracks. The smooth surface keeps everything right where you want it. If you weren't already a burger lover, your gas griddle might just change your mind.

TIPS FOR MAKING BURGERS ON A GAS GRIDDLE

- Use a combo of 80/20 ground beef. That extra fat is what keeps your patties juicy.
- Don't overcrowd the griddle. Cook your patties in batches if you have to. You need room to work.
- For the love of all that is holy, do not start mashing down on the patties with your spatula once they're cooking. That'll just squeeze out all the good juices.
- Flip your patties just once during cooking. Any more flipping, and you'll dry them out.
- Make your own burger seasoning blend with dried herbs, spices, and a little brown sugar.
- Use your thumb to make a shallow indent in the center of each raw patty. This helps them cook evenly and prevent puffing.
- Chill the formed patties in the fridge for 30 minutes before cooking. This helps them hold their shape better on the griddle.
- Use a melting dome to speed up the cheese-melting process for thick cheeseburgers. The dome traps heat and steam to help the cheese melt faster.
- If you're new to griddle cooking, be prepared for how quickly everything happens. Prep all your ingredients in advance to avoid getting caught off guard.
- Aim for a griddle temperature between 375-450°F when cooking your patties.
- Be careful of splattering grease when cooking burgers on the griddle. Since the flat surface doesn't allow the fat to escape, thinner patties, in particular, can cause the grease to splatter upwards.

KITCHEN TOOLS NEEDED

- Melting dome
- Potato masher
- Saucepan
- Basting brush
- Mixing bowls
- Aluminum foil
- Cutting board
- Food processor
- Wire rack
- Oven (to make your own burger buns)

CLASSIC BEEF BURGER

Serving: 4
Prep time: 10 mins
Cooking time: 20 mins

INGREDIENTS:

- 1 lb. ground beef
- 4 teaspoons of salt
- 2 teaspoons of black pepper
- 4 brioche or potato burger buns, split in half

- 4 slices of American cheese
- 8 tablespoons of butter, divided
- Toppings of your choice (lettuce, tomato, onion, pickles, etc.)

DIRECTIONS:

1. Form ¼ of the ground beef into a 4-inch wide, 1-inch thick patty. Season both sides generously with salt and pepper.

2. Preheat your gas griddle on medium-high heat. Drop 1 tablespoon of the butter onto the surface and let it melt.

3. Carefully place the beef patty on the hot griddle. Cook for 4 to 5 minutes per side until it reaches your desired doneness. During the last minute of cooking, top the patty with a slice of cheese so it can melt.

4. While the burger is cooking, melt another tablespoon of butter on the griddle and toast 1 of the bun halves until golden brown.

5. Transfer the cheeseburger patty to the toasted bun bottom. Top with your favorite toppings and the top bun. Follow these steps to make more burgers.

6. Instead of the classic French fries, serve with grilled vegetables this time.

BACON CHEESEBURGER

Serving: 4
Prep time: 10 mins
Cooking time: 20 mins

INGREDIENTS:

- 1 lb. ground beef
- 4 teaspoons of salt
- 2 teaspoons of black pepper
- 8 slices of bacon
- 4 slice of cheddar cheese
- 4 brioche buns, split in half
- 4 tablespoons of butter, divided

DIRECTIONS:

1. Shape your beef into 4 patties and season both sides with salt and pepper.
2. Preheat your gas griddle on medium-high heat. Place 2 tablespoons of butter on the hot surface for it to melt.
3. Place the bacon slices on the hot griddle and cook until crispy, about 2 to 3 minutes per side. Transfer the cooked bacon to a paper towel-lined plate.
4. Add the beef patty to the griddle and cook for 4 to 5 minutes per side or until it reaches your preferred doneness. Top the patty with a slice of cheddar cheese a minute before you take it off the griddle.
5. While the burger cooks, drop the remaining butter on the griddle and toast the bun halves.
6. Transfer the cheeseburger patty to the toasted bun bottom. Top with the bacon slices, and close the burger with the top bun half.
7. This will go beautifully with mac and cheese.

CHICKPEA FALAFEL BURGER (VEGAN)

Serving: 2
Prep time: 15 mins
Cooking time: 15 mins

INGREDIENTS:

- 1 cup of cooked chickpeas (garbanzo beans), drained and patted dry
- 4 tablespoons of finely chopped onion
- 2 minced garlic cloves
- 2 teaspoons of ground cumin
- 1 teaspoon of ground coriander
- ½ teaspoon of cayenne pepper

- 3 tablespoons of all-purpose flour
- 2 tablespoons of olive oil, plus more for cooking
- Salt and pepper for seasoning
- 2 burger buns, split in half
- Toppings like tomato, cucumber, red onion, tahini sauce (optional)

DIRECTIONS:

1. Mash the chickpeas with a fork or potato masher until you get a chunky paste. Stir in the onion, garlic, cumin, coriander, cayenne, flour, and 1 tablespoon of olive oil. Season with salt and pepper.
2. Shape ½ of the chickpea mixture into a patty about 4 inches wide and a half-inch thick.
3. Heat your gas griddle on medium-high and spread a thin layer of olive oil over the surface.
4. Carefully place the falafel patty on the hot griddle. Cook for 3 to 4 minutes per side or until it is golden brown.
5. While the falafel cooks, toast the bun halves on the griddle.
6. Transfer the hot falafel patty to the bottom bun. Top with your favorites like tomato, cucumber, red onion, and a drizzle of tahini sauce if you'd like.
7. Close up your falafel burger and serve with your favorite salad.

LAMB KOFTA BURGER

Serving: 2
Prep time: 10 mins
Cooking time: 20 mins

INGREDIENTS:

- ½ lb. ground lamb
- 2 tablespoons of finely chopped onion
- 2 minced garlic cloves
- 2 teaspoons of ground cumin
- 1 teaspoon of ground coriander
- ½ teaspoon of cayenne pepper
- Salt and pepper for seasoning
- 2 brioche buns, split in half
- Toppings like tzatziki sauce, tomato, yellow onion, lettuce (optional)

DIRECTIONS:

1. Mix the ground lamb, onion, garlic, cumin, coriander, and cayenne in a bowl. Sprinkle salt and pepper and mix again. Shape ½ of the mixture into a patty.
2. Preheat your gas griddle on medium-high heat and add a drizzle of oil to the surface.
3. Place the lamb kofta patty onto the hot griddle. Cook for 4 to 5 minutes per side until the outside is nicely browned and the inside is cooked through.
4. While the kofta burger is cooking, toast your bun halves on the griddle until crisp.
5. Transfer the cooked kofta patty to the bottom bun. Top with tzatziki sauce, fresh tomato slices, yellow onion, and lettuce leaves.
6. Close up your lamb kofta burger and serve.

LENTIL AND QUINOA BURGER (VEGAN)

Serving: 2
Prep time: 10 mins
Cooking time: 15 mins

INGREDIENTS:

- ½ lb. cooked lentils
- 4 tablespoons of cooked quinoa
- 2 tablespoons of finely chopped onion
- 2 minced garlic cloves
- 1 teaspoon of ground cumin
- ½ teaspoon of smoked paprika
- 4 tablespoons of breadcrumbs

- 2 tablespoons of olive oil, plus more for cooking
- Salt and black pepper for seasoning
- 2 whole wheat burger buns, split in half
- Sliced avocado
- Roasted red pepper
- Sprouts or greens

DIRECTIONS:

1. Get a medium bowl and mash the cooked lentils until they're chunky. Pour in the cooked quinoa, onion, garlic, cumin, smoked paprika, breadcrumbs, and 1 tablespoon of olive oil. Season the mixture with salt and pepper.
2. Shape the lentil-quinoa blend into 2 patties.
3. Heat your gas griddle on medium and pour a light coating of oil on the surface.
4. Place the lentil-quinoa patties onto the hot griddle and cook for 4 to 5 minutes per side until the exterior is crispy and properly browned.
5. While the burger cooks, toast the whole wheat bun halves on the griddle.
6. Once the lentil-quinoa patties are cooked through, place 1 on a bottom bun and top with sliced avocado, roasted red pepper, sprouts, or any other toppings you like.
7. Close it and serve with garlic-yogurt dipping sauce.

BUFFALO CHICKEN BURGER

Serving: 2
Prep time: 10 mins
Cooking time: 25 mins

INGREDIENTS:

- 8 ounces of ground chicken
- 4 tablespoons of buffalo wing sauce
- 2 tablespoons of breadcrumbs
- 2 eggs
- ½ teaspoon of garlic powder
- ½ teaspoon of onion powder
- A pinch of smoked paprika

- A pinch of salt
- A pinch of black pepper
- 2 burger buns
- 2 slices of cheddar cheese (optional)
- 2 tablespoons of shredded lettuce
- 4 tomato slices

DIRECTIONS:

1. Preheat your gas griddle on medium-high heat.
2. Mix the ground chicken, buffalo sauce, breadcrumbs, egg, garlic powder, onion powder, smoked paprika, salt, and pepper in a bowl.
3. Gently form the chicken mixture into 2 patties. Try not to overwork the meat.
4. Place the patties on the hot griddle and cook for 5 to 6 minutes per side until it reaches 165°F inside. Add the cheese slice on top during the last minute if you'll be using it.
5. While the burgers are cooking, toast your bun halves on the griddle.
6. Put 1 chicken patty on the bottom bun, then top with the shredded lettuce and tomato slices. Close it with the top bun. Do the same for the other burger.
7. Serve right away, with extra buffalo sauce on the side for dipping if you like.

SMOKEY TEMPEH BURGER (VEGAN)

Serving: 2
Prep time: 5 mins
Cooking time: 15 mins

INGREDIENTS:

- 1 lb. tempeh, crumbled
- 4 tablespoons of soy sauce
- 2 tablespoons of smoked paprika
- 2 tablespoons of olive oil
- 2 teaspoons of maple syrup
- ½ teaspoon of garlic powder
- ½ teaspoon of onion powder

- A pinch of cayenne pepper
- A pinch of salt
- A pinch of black pepper
- 2 burger buns, halved
- 2 slices of vegan cheddar cheese (optional)
- 4 tablespoons of shredded cabbage
- 2 tablespoon of sliced pickles

DIRECTIONS:

1. Preheat your gas griddle on medium heat.
2. Mix the crumbled tempeh, soy sauce, smoked paprika, olive oil, maple syrup, garlic powder, onion powder, cayenne, salt, and pepper in a bowl.
3. Scoop the tempeh mixture and shape it into 2 patties. Handle it gently to keep the texture.
4. Place the tempeh patties on the preheated griddle. Cook for 5 to 6 minutes per side until it's browned. Now is the time to add the cheese slice on top if you are using it.
5. While the patty cooks, toast your bun on the griddle.
6. Place 1 cooked tempeh patty on a bottom bun. Top with the shredded cabbage and sliced pickles. Close it with the top bun, and serve.

TERIYAKI CHICKEN BURGERS

Serving: 4
Prep time: 15 mins
Cooking time: 25 mins

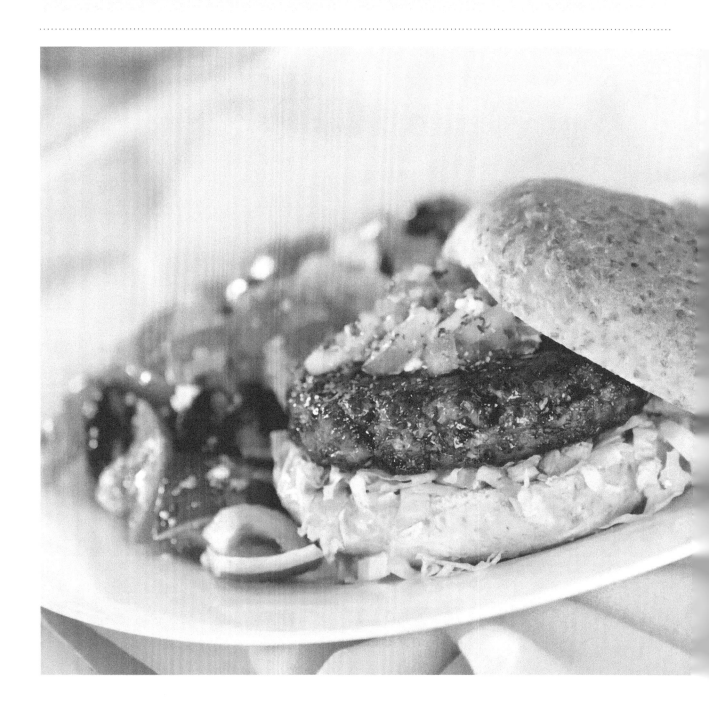

INGREDIENTS:

- 1 lb. ground chicken
- 2 tablespoons of soy sauce
- 1 tablespoon of brown sugar
- 1 tablespoon of rice vinegar
- 1 teaspoon of sesame oil
- 1 teaspoon of grated ginger
- 1 teaspoon of grated garlic
- ½ teaspoon of ground black pepper
- 4 brioche burger buns, split

- Butter, for the griddle
- 4 slices of cheddar cheese (optional)

Teriyaki Glaze:

- ¼ cup of soy sauce
- 2 tablespoons of brown sugar
- 1 tablespoon of rice vinegar
- 1 teaspoon of sesame oil
- ½ teaspoon of ground ginger

DIRECTIONS:

1. Make the teriyaki glaze first. Whisk the soy sauce, brown sugar, rice vinegar, sesame oil, and ground ginger in a saucepan. Bring it to a simmer over medium heat and leave it for 2 to 3 minutes until it thickens. Turn off the heat and set the pan aside.

2. Grab a large bowl and mix the ground chicken, soy sauce, brown sugar, rice vinegar, sesame oil, grated ginger, grated garlic, and black pepper. Mix everything very gently.

3. Preheat your gas griddle on medium-high heat and butter the surface.

4. Divide the chicken mixture into 4 equal portions and shape into patties.

5. Cook the patties on the griddle for 4 to 5 minutes per side or until they are cooked to your liking.

6. Right at the last minute, brush the patties with the teriyaki glaze and top with a slice of cheddar cheese if you'll be using it.

7. Toast the brioche buns while the patties get ready.

8. Place the teriyaki chicken patties on the bottom buns. Top with your preferred toppings, then add the top buns and serve with a macaroni salad on the side.

MAPLE DIJON SALMON BURGER

Serving: 4
Prep time: 15 mins
Cooking time: 25 mins

INGREDIENTS:

- 1 lb. fresh salmon filet, skin removed and shaped into 4 patties
- 2 tablespoons of maple syrup
- 2 tablespoons of Dijon mustard
- 1 teaspoon of garlic powder
- 1 teaspoon of onion powder
- ½ teaspoon of salt
- ¼ teaspoon of black pepper
- 4 brioche buns, split in half
- Butter or olive oil
- Optional toppings: lettuce, tomato, red onion, cheese, etc.

DIRECTIONS:

1. Grab a shallow bowl and mix the maple syrup, Dijon mustard, garlic powder, onion powder, salt, and pepper.
2. Dunk the salmon patties in the mixture, ensuring they're coated on both sides.
3. Preheat your gas griddle to medium-high and give it a light grease with butter or olive oil.
4. Gently place the salmon patties on the hot griddle and cook them for 4 to 5 minutes on each side until they're cooked through and flaky.
5. While the salmon is cooking, place the brioche buns, cut side down, on the griddle until they're toasted.
6. Assemble your burgers by placing a salmon patty on the bottom bun, followed by your favorite toppings, and then capping it off with the top bun.

SPICY CHILE BURGER

Serving: 2
Prep time: 15 mins
Cooking time: 30 mins

INGREDIENTS:

- 1 lbs. ground beef chuck
- ½ teaspoon of black pepper
- 1 chipotle pepper in adobo sauce, chopped, plus 2 teaspoons of the sauce
- 2 tablespoons of mayonnaise
- 1 teaspoon of kosher salt
- 4 slices of Pepper Jack or Pepper Colby cheese
- 2 burger buns
- 2 fresh poblano or hatch chiles
- 2 tablespoons of sliced pickled jalapeños

DIRECTIONS:

1. Season the ground beef with salt and pepper. Gently shape the beef into two patties.
2. Put your gas griddle on high. Place the whole chiles directly on the hot surface and let them blacken and blister. This should take about 5 to 7 minutes.
3. Once the chiles are charred, transfer them to a bowl and cover tightly with foil. Let them steam for 5 minutes to loosen up the skins. Then, peel off and discard the charred skins.
4. Mix the chopped chipotle pepper, the adobo sauce, and the mayonnaise in a small bowl. This will be your spicy mayo to top the burgers.
5. Your griddle should still be hot from step 2. Turn the knob to medium and grease the surface with a bit of oil or butter.
6. Add the burger patties and cook each side for 4 to 5 minutes or until they're seared and cooked to your liking. At the last minute, top each patty with 2 slices of cheese.
7. While the burgers are cooking, toast the buns on the griddle.
8. Place a patty on the bottom bun, then top with the roasted chiles, pickled jalapeños, and a big dollop of the chipotle mayo. Cover with the top bun and serve.
9. This will go well with the grilled potato salad with bacon vinaigrette from pg. 178.

CAJUN AND REMOULADE BURGER

Serving: 2
Prep time: 30 mins
Cooking time: 10 mins

INGREDIENTS:

- ½ lb. ground beef chuck
- 4 ounces of Creole andouille sausage, diced into ½-inch pieces
- ½ cup of mayonnaise
- 2 tablespoons of Dijon mustard
- 2 teaspoons of lemon juice
- 2 teaspoons of ketchup
- ¼ white onion, thinly sliced
- ½ teaspoon of cayenne pepper
- ½ large red bell pepper, thinly sliced

- 2 teaspoons of prepared horseradish
- 2 teaspoons of hot sauce (e.g., Tabasco)
- 2 minced garlic cloves
- Salt and pepper for seasoning
- 2 celery stalk, peeled into thin strips
- Vegetable oil for brushing
- 2 burger buns
- 2 teaspoons of chopped fresh parsley
- 4 ounces of crumbled blue cheese

DIRECTIONS:

1. Use a small food processor to blend the beef and andouille sausage until they're coarsely mixed, then shape them into 2 patties that are a bit bigger than the buns. Make a small dimple in the center, and then place it in the fridge until you're ready to cook it.
2. Use the same processor to make the remoulade sauce by blending mayo, ketchup, hot sauce, mustard, parsley, lemon juice, cayenne, horseradish, and garlic until smooth. Don't forget to season it with salt and pepper before setting it aside.
3. Put the celery strips in ice water and keep them in the fridge for later.
4. Preheat your gas griddle to medium-high. Brush oil on the onion and bell pepper slices and cook them for about 4 minutes until they're charred.
5. Remove your burger patties from the fridge and sprinkle it with salt and pepper.
6. Throw them onto the griddle for 3 to 4 minutes per side or until they're cooked just the way you like it.
7. While the burger is cooking, toast the buns on the griddle.
8. To assemble your burger, put 1 patty on the bottom bun and top it with the remoulade, the grilled onions and peppers, the celery strips, and the crumbled blue cheese. Place the top bun on and serve.

SMASH CHEESEBURGER

Serving: 2
Prep time: 5 mins
Cooking time: 5 mins

INGREDIENTS:

- 2 burger buns, split in half
- 8 ounces of ground beef chuck, split into two 2-ounce portions
- Kosher salt and ground black pepper
- 2 slices of any good melting cheese (like American, cheddar, etc.)
- Favorite toppings and condiments (mayo, mustard, lettuce, onion, tomato, pickles, etc.)

DIRECTIONS:

1. Put your gas griddle on high heat and let it preheat for a couple of minutes.
2. Once the griddle is a little hot, toast your burger bun. Set the prepared bun aside, ready to go.
3. Take your two beef balls and place them on the hot griddle. Press down firmly on each one using a sturdy spatula to smash them into thin, wide patties. Sprinkle each one with salt and pepper.
4. Let them sizzle for about 2 minutes or until they're well-browned on the bottom and just starting to turn a pale gray color on top.
5. Carefully scrape the smashed patties off the griddle with a spatula or bench scraper, making sure to get all those browned bits.
6. Immediately, place the slice of cheese on top of one of the patties, then quickly stack the other patty right on top. The residual heat will melt the cheese.
7. Transfer the stacked, cheesy smash burger onto the waiting toasted bun bottom.
8. Top with your favorite toppings and condiments, and cover with the bun lid.
9. Serve with fries and lemon wedges.

BRIOCHE BURGER BUNS

Serving: 8
Prep time: 1 hr 45 mins
Cooking time: 18 mins

INGREDIENTS:

- 2¼ teaspoon (1 packet) of active dry yeast
- ¼ cup of warm water (110-115°F)
- ¼ cup of granulated sugar
- 1 cup of whole milk, warmed to 110-115°F
- 2 large eggs at room temperature
- 1 teaspoon of salt
- 4 cups of all-purpose flour, plus more for dusting
- 6 tablespoons of unsalted butter, softened

DIRECTIONS:

1. Pour the warm water, yeast, and 1 teaspoon of sugar into a bowl. Let it sit for 5 to 10 minutes until you see foam at the top.
2. Warm the milk over medium heat until it reaches 110 to 115°F. Take it off the heat and stir in the remaining sugar until it dissolves. Leave it to cool a little bit.
3. Get another bowl and whisk the eggs and salt.
4. Add the yeast, warm milk, and 2 cups of flour to the egg mixture. Use a wooden spoon or strong spatula to mix everything until a shaggy dough forms.
5. Turn the dough out onto a lightly floured surface and knead for about 5 minutes, working in the remaining 2 cups of flour until the dough is smooth, elastic, and not too sticky.
6. Place the dough in a large, greased bowl. Cover and leave it to rise in a warm place for 1 hour or until it doubles in size.
7. Punch down the dough to release any air bubbles. Turn it onto a floured surface and knead in the softened butter for 2 to 3 minutes.
8. Divide the dough into 8 equal pieces. Shape each piece into a smooth ball. Place the balls on a parchment-lined baking sheet with a few inches between each ball.
9. Cover the buns and let them rise for 30 minutes.
10. Preheat the oven to 400°F.
11. Bake for 15 to 18 minutes until the tops are golden brown.
12. Let the buns cool completely on a wire rack before slicing and using.

Chapter 6:
Pasta and Italian

Statistics tells us that the average person in the United States eats over 20 pounds of pasta per year, which puts into perspective just how much pasta is collectively consumed as a society.

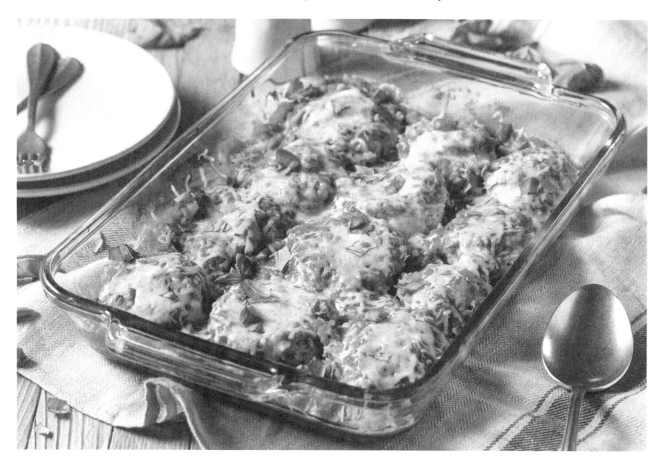

That's a staggering amount when you think about it. If you break it down, 20 pounds of pasta is the equivalent of over 10,000 individual strands. That's a lot of slurping and twirling of forks to get through that much pasta over a year. And to think, that's just the average. Plenty of pasta lovers out there blow that number out of the water. Clearly, pasta is a favorite for so many people that they probably don't even realize how much of it they're eating regularly.

Cooking pasta on a gas griddle is actually really clever and versatile. One major benefit is the ability to multitask. You can boil your pasta on one section of the griddle while simultaneously sautéing vegetables or simmering a sauce on another part. You need a large enough griddle surface to accommodate the pasta pot and any other prep work you need to do. With the amount of pasta the average American consumes, that kind of efficiency in the kitchen is a dream. Pasta may be a simple pleasure, but it deserves to be celebrated, and that means doing whatever it takes to make it as easy and enjoyable as possible.

TIPS FOR MAKING PASTA ON A GAS GRIDDLE

- Add a splash of pasta cooking water to the griddle surface occasionally to create steam and prevent the pasta from sticking.

- Keep the griddle surface clean between batches to prevent sticking.
- If you don't have a side burner, you can boil the pasta on your gas griddle top. Place a pot of water directly on the preheated griddle set to medium-high heat.
- Your pasta will continue to cook a bit more once removed from the heat, so you'll want to pull it from the water just shy of being fully al dente.

KITCHEN TOOLS NEEDED

- Any metal pot
- Stovetop (This is optional because you can place the pot of water directly on the hot griddle)
- Serving plates

PASTA WITH TOMATO AND BASIL

Serving: 4
Prep time: 10 mins
Cooking time: 25 mins

INGREDIENTS:

- 8 ounces of dried spaghetti or linguine pasta
- 3 tablespoons of olive oil
- 4 minced cloves of garlic
- 1 (28 oz) can of diced tomatoes
- 1 teaspoon of dried oregano
- ¼ teaspoon of red pepper flakes (optional)
- ½ cup of fresh basil leaves, chopped
- Salt and black pepper for seasoning
- Grated Parmesan cheese for serving (optional)

DIRECTIONS:

1. Bring a pot of salted water to a boil on your stovetop or one side of your griddle surface. Add the dried pasta and cook until al dente. Drain the cooked pasta and set it aside.
2. Heat your olive oil on the preheated griddle over medium heat.
3. Add the minced garlic to the hot oil and cook for 1 minute, stirring until you can smell the garlic.
4. Pour the can of diced tomatoes and their juices directly onto the griddle. Add the oregano and red pepper flakes (if using). Season with a pinch of salt and pepper.
5. Give the tomato sauce time to simmer for 5 to 7 minutes or until it thickens a bit.
6. Pour the cooked pasta into the tomato sauce and toss to coat the strands thoroughly.
7. Turn off the heat and stir in the chopped basil.
8. Serve the pasta immediately, right off the griddle. Top with grated Parmesan cheese for extra flavor.

CHICKEN PASTA PRIMAVERA

Serving: 4
Prep time: 10 mins
Cooking time: 35 mins

INGREDIENTS:

- 8 ounces of dried farfalle (bowtie) pasta
- 2 boneless, skinless chicken breasts, cubed
- 2 tablespoons of olive oil
- 2 minced cloves of garlic
- 1 red bell pepper, sliced
- 1 zucchini, sliced
- 1 cup of broccoli florets
- 1 cup of cherry tomatoes, halved
- ½ cup of heavy cream
- ¼ cup of grated Parmesan cheese
- 2 tablespoons of chopped fresh basil
- Salt and black pepper for seasoning

DIRECTIONS:

1. Cook the pasta in salted water on your stovetop. Drain and set aside.
2. Heat olive oil on the griddle preheated over medium heat. Add the cubed chicken and sauté until it is cooked through, about 6 to 8 minutes. Depending on the size of your griddle, you can move the chicken to a plate or go to another section of the griddle to cook the other ingredients simultaneously.
3. On the same griddle, sauté the garlic for 1 minute until it is fragrant. Add the sliced bell pepper, zucchini, and broccoli. Cook for 4 to 5 minutes. Don't forget to stir.
4. Pour the heavy cream onto the griddle and let it simmer for 2 to 3 minutes. Stir until you see it thicken.
5. Add the cooked chicken, cherry tomatoes, Parmesan cheese, and chopped basil. Toss everything together on the griddle.
6. Finally, add the cooked farfalle pasta and toss again to coat everything.
7. Season with salt and pepper, and serve garnished with extra basil.

SHRIMP PASTA WITH LEMON AND GARLIC

Serving: 4
Prep time: 10 mins
Cooking time: 25 mins

INGREDIENTS:

- 8 ounces of dried linguine pasta
- 1 lb. large shrimp, peeled and deveined
- 3 tablespoons of olive oil
- 4 minced cloves of garlic
- ½ cup of dry white wine

- Zest and juice of 1 lemon
- ¼ cup of chopped fresh parsley
- Salt and black pepper for seasoning
- Grated Parmesan cheese for serving (optional)

DIRECTIONS:

1. Boil the pasta on the stovetop. When it reaches al dente, drain the water and set it aside.

2. In the meantime, preheat your griddle to medium-high. Drizzle some olive oil on the hot surface, and add the minced garlic. Sauté for 1 minute.

3. Add the shrimp to the griddle and cook for 2 to 3 minutes per side until they are opaque and cooked through. Transfer the sautéed shrimp to a plate.

4. Pour the white wine directly onto the hot griddle, scraping any browned bits from the shrimp. Let it simmer for 1 or 2 minutes.

5. Reduce the heat to low and return the cooked shrimp to the griddle. Stir in the lemon zest and juice. Sprinkle salt and pepper over it.

6. Add the cooked linguine and chopped parsley. Toss everything until the pasta is heated through and coated in the lemon-garlic sauce. Serve with grated Parmesan cheese if you like.

CREAMY CAJUN CHICKEN PASTA

Serving: 2
Prep time: 10 mins
Cooking time: 20 mins

INGREDIENTS:

- 4 ounces of dry penne pasta
- 1 boneless, skinless chicken thigh, cubed
- 1 tablespoon of olive oil
- 2 teaspoons of Cajun seasoning
- 2 tablespoons of unsalted butter
- 2 tablespoons of heavy cream
- 2 tablespoons of shredded Parmesan cheese
- 2 tablespoons of diced tomatoes
- 1 tablespoon of chopped fresh parsley
- Salt and black pepper for seasoning

DIRECTIONS:

1. Cook the penne pasta. When it is ready, drain it and set it aside.

2. Meanwhile, preheat your griddle on medium-high heat. Coat the cubed chicken thigh with the Cajun seasoning, then pour it onto the hot griddle surface and sauté. The chicken should be cooked through in roughly 5 to 6 minutes.

3. While that happens, melt the butter on another section of the griddle if you have enough space. Once it is completely melted, stir in the heavy cream. Allow the creamy sauce to simmer for 1 or 2 minutes. It should look thick at the end of this.

4. Turn the heat to low and stir the cooked chicken into the creamy sauce. Add the drained penne pasta and toss to coat the pasta.

5. Sprinkle the shredded Parmesan cheese over the top, then diced tomatoes and fresh parsley. Sprinkle salt and pepper. Toss again and serve.

ITALIAN CUISINE

Italians have a deep respect for quality ingredients and a commitment to simplicity. They know that when you start with the best, you don't need to do too much to make something great, and that is the most straightforward definition of Italian cuisine you'll probably get.

Now, can you make Italian food on a gas griddle? Absolutely. Paninis, frittatas, and quick-seared meats work great on the griddle, but some classic Italian recipes, like slow-cooked ragus or wood-fired pizzas, may not translate so well. You might not be able to replicate that wood-fired pizza crust accurately, but it doesn't matter when you can get creative and make something new. If you can adapt the recipes to your equipment, you can cook almost anything. Here are some recipes to get you inspired.

TIPS FOR MAKING ITALIAN FOOD ON A GAS GRIDDLE

- Start with the highest quality, freshest ingredients you can find, from extra virgin olive oil to Parmigiano-Reggiano cheese.
- Get familiar with Italian cuisine's core spices and seasonings, such as oregano, basil, rosemary, garlic, and red pepper flakes.
- Use the griddle to toast bread crumbs or panko for breading or topping dishes.
- Season as you go. Your meals can turn out however you want, but only if you take control of the seasoning process.

KITCHEN TOOLS NEEDED

- Basting brush
- Mixing bowls
- Serving plates

EGGPLANT PARMESAN STACKS

Serving: 4
Prep time: 10 mins
Cooking time: 15 mins

INGREDIENTS:

- 2 medium eggplants, sliced into ½-inch thick rounds (about 12 to 15 slices per eggplant)
- 2 tablespoons of olive oil
- Salt and pepper for seasoning
- 1 cup of marinara sauce
- 1½ cups of shredded mozzarella cheese

DIRECTIONS:

1. Brush both sides of the eggplant slices with a little olive oil and season them with salt and pepper.
2. Place the eggplant slices directly on the hot griddle. Cook for 3 to 4 minutes on both sides.
3. Once the eggplant is ready, it's time to build your stacks. Place one grilled eggplant slice on a plate, then top with a couple of tablespoons of marinara sauce and a sprinkle of mozzarella cheese. Repeat this process, stacking the eggplant slices with the marinara and cheese between each layer.
4. Keep going until you've used up all your grilled eggplant slices. You should end up with 4 or 5 stacks.
5. Place the assembled stacks back on the griddle for 2 to 3 minutes until the cheese melts and is bubbly on top.
6. Serve warm, with tomato and basil pasta (Pg. 73) if you're ready to fall in love with a meal.

BRUSCHETTA

Serving: 8
Prep time: 15 mins
Cooking time: 10 mins

INGREDIENTS:

- 1 baguette or crusty Italian bread, sliced into ¼-inch thick slices
- 3 tablespoons of olive oil, plus more for brushing
- 3 minced cloves of garlic
- 2 cups of diced tomatoes
- ¼ cup of chopped fresh basil
- 2 tablespoons of balsamic vinegar
- ¼ teaspoon of salt
- ¼ teaspoon of black pepper
- ½ cup of shredded or crumbled mozzarella or parmesan cheese (optional)

DIRECTIONS:

1. Preheat your griddle over medium-high heat.
2. Into a medium bowl, pour the olive oil and garlic. Let that sit for 2 or 3 minutes to infuse the oil with garlic flavor.
3. Brush both sides of the bread slices lightly with the extra olive oil.
4. Place the oiled bread slices directly on the hot griddle. Toast for 2 to 3 minutes per side until golden brown and crispy. Transfer the toasted bread to a plate when it's done.
5. While that is happening, add the diced tomatoes, basil, balsamic vinegar, salt, and pepper to the garlic-infused olive oil. Stir to combine.
6. Top each toasted bread slice with a spoonful of the tomato-basil mixture. If you want to, sprinkle a bit of mozzarella or parmesan cheese over the top.
7. Serve the bruschetta immediately while the bread is still warm and crispy. Grilled vegetables on the side are always a good choice.

PASTA WITH ROASTED GARLIC ALFREDO

Serving: 2
Prep time: 5 mins
Cooking time: 35 mins

INGREDIENTS:

- 3 ounces of dried fettuccine pasta
- 1 small head of garlic
- 2 tablespoons of unsalted butter
- ¼ cup of heavy cream
- ¼ cup of grated Parmesan cheese
- 1 tablespoon of chopped fresh parsley
- Salt and black pepper for seasoning

DIRECTIONS:

1. Preheat your griddle on medium-high heat.
2. Take the small head of garlic and slice the top off to expose the cloves. Place the whole head directly on the hot griddle surface and roast for 15 to 20 minutes. Turn it occasionally until it is soft and fragrant. Remove the roasted garlic from the griddle and set it aside.
3. While the garlic is roasting, add the fettuccine pasta to boiling salted water and cook per package directions. Drain the cooked pasta and set it aside.
4. Bring a small bowl and gently squeeze the roasted garlic cloves to extract the soft, creamy paste. You should have about 1 to 2 tablespoons of roasted garlic in there.
5. Place the butter on the griddle. Once it is melted, whisk in the heavy cream and the roasted garlic paste. Leave the sauce to simmer for 1 to 2 minutes until it looks thickened.
6. Reduce the heat to low and stir in the grated Parmesan cheese until it is melted and the sauce is smooth and creamy.
7. Add the cooked fettuccine to the alfredo sauce and toss until the pasta is fully coated in the garlicky sauce.
8. Take it off the heat and stir in chopped fresh parsley. Sprinkle with salt and pepper, and serve.

CHICKEN CACCIATORE

Serving: 4
Prep time: 10 mins
Cooking time: 30 mins

INGREDIENTS:

- 1.5 lbs. boneless, skinless chicken breasts or thighs cut into 1-inch pieces
- 1 teaspoon of salt
- 1 teaspoon of black pepper
- 1 teaspoon of garlic powder
- 1 onion, diced

- 1 red bell pepper, diced
- 1 (28oz) can of crushed tomatoes
- ½ cup of red wine
- ½ cup of chicken stock
- ½ cup of kalamata olives, sliced (optional)

DIRECTIONS:

1. Preheat your griddle to medium.
2. Put the chicken pieces in a bowl, and season them with salt, pepper, and garlic powder. Make sure each little chunk is thoroughly coated.
3. With the griddle raging hot, go ahead and add the seasoned chicken. Let them cook for a minute or two before flipping.
4. Once the chicken is browned, push it to one side of the griddle and add the diced onions and bell peppers. Sauté the vegetables for a few minutes until they soften.
5. Mix the sautéed vegetables and the chicken. Pour in the crushed tomatoes, red wine, and chicken stock. Stir properly.
6. Let that simmer on the griddle, stirring periodically, until the sauce is thick and the chicken is cooked through, about 15 to 20 minutes.
7. For a bit of flair, add the sliced olives at the end. Serve with a side of pasta or some garlic bread.

Chapter 7:
Fusion Meals and International Flavors

In the simplest terms, fusion meals are a mash-up of different types of cuisine into one dish. You take your favorite flavors from around the world and combine them however you think will make sense.

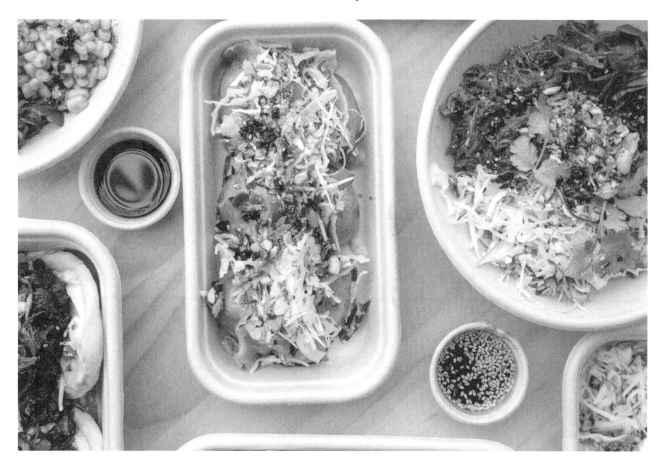

Fusion cooking started to take off in the 1970s, as people had more access to ingredients and cooking techniques from different cultures. Chefs and home cooks started experimenting, blending spices, seasonings, and cooking methods from as many traditions as they could. The goal was to create bold, complex flavors that you wouldn't find in a traditional dish. The features of this cooking style are:

- Using ingredients or cooking styles from multiple cuisines in one dish.
- Putting a fresh spin on classic recipes by adding unexpected elements.
- Focusing on big, interesting flavors and fun flavor combinations.
- Presentation that mixes visual styles from different culinary traditions.
- Flexibility to swap in different ingredients based on what's available.

Now imagine all that but on a griddle. The griddle is the perfect canvas for fusion cooking. All you have to think about is how the different elements will complement each other. Do you want to marinate some chicken in a Thai-inspired sauce, then top it with a Latin American-style salsa and some toasted peanuts? Done. Or you could start with a base of hash browns, then layer on Korean-style bulgogi, kimchi, and a runny fried egg. You can do almost anything on a griddle. Have fun, and don't be afraid to experiment. Mix and match ingredients, cooking methods, and presentation styles to your heart's content. If you need some inspiration, here are a few popular fusion recipes.

TIPS FOR MAKING FUSION MEALS ON A GRIDDLE

- Start with the aromatic all-stars—ginger, garlic, scallions—to build a killer flavor base.
- Use the right high-heat oils for stir-frying to avoid burning.
- Create signature fusion sauces by mixing the classics, e.g., soy sauce, mirin, and gochujang.
- Use a combination of proteins—chicken, shrimp, tofu—for textural contrast in your stir-fries.
- Use your griddle's cool zones to keep sauces and garnishes warm while cooking proteins.

KITCHEN TOOLS NEEDED

- Mixing bowls
- Serving plates

KOREAN BBQ BEEF STIR-FRY

Serving: 2
Prep time: 20 mins
Cooking time: 10 mins

INGREDIENTS:

- 6 ounces of flank steak, thinly sliced against the grain
- 2 tablespoons of soy sauce
- 1 tablespoon of brown sugar
- 1 tablespoon of sesame oil
- 2 minced cloves of garlic
- 1 teaspoon of grated fresh ginger
- ½ teaspoon of red pepper flakes

- 1 cup of kimchi, chopped
- 1 cup of bean sprouts
- 1 tablespoon of gochujang (Korean red chili paste)
- 1 tablespoon of vegetable oil
- 1 cup of cooked white rice for serving
- Toasted sesame seeds, for garnish
- Sliced green onions for garnish

DIRECTIONS:

1. Preheat your griddle on medium–high heat.
2. Put the sliced flank steak, soy sauce, brown sugar, sesame oil, garlic, ginger, and red pepper flakes in a small bowl. Coat the beef with the marinade and let it marinate for 10 minutes.
3. Pour the vegetable oil on the hot griddle surface and follow with the marinated beef. Stir-fry for 3 to 4 minutes, until it is just cooked through. Transfer the beef to a plate for later.
4. Without cleaning the griddle, add the chopped kimchi and bean sprouts. Stir-fry for 2 to 3 minutes, until the kimchi is soft and the bean sprouts are soft yet crisp.
5. Push the kimchi and bean sprouts to one side of the griddle. Add the gochujang paste to the empty space and let it sizzle for 30 seconds, then stir it into the vegetables.
6. Return the cooked beef to the griddle and toss everything properly.
7. Serve your stir-fry over a bed of cooked white rice. Garnish with toasted sesame seeds and sliced green onions.

THAI PEANUT CHICKEN STIR-FRY

Serving: 2
Prep time: 20 mins
Cooking time: 10 mins

INGREDIENTS:

- 6 ounces of boneless, skinless chicken thighs cut into 1-inch pieces
- 2 tablespoons of soy sauce
- 1 tablespoon of brown sugar
- 1 tablespoon of fish sauce
- 1 teaspoon of red curry paste
- 1 tablespoon of vegetable oil
- ½ red bell pepper, sliced

- ½ cup of snow peas, trimmed
- 2 tablespoons of creamy peanut butter
- 2 tablespoons of coconut milk
- 1 tablespoon of lime juice
- ¼ cup of chopped roasted peanuts
- Chopped fresh cilantro for garnish
- Cooked jasmine rice for serving

DIRECTIONS:

1. Preheat your griddle over medium-high heat.
2. Mix the cubed chicken, soy sauce, brown sugar, fish sauce, and red curry paste in a bowl. Make sure the chicken is thoroughly coated, and leave it to marinate for 8 to 10 minutes.
3. Drizzle the vegetable oil on the griddle surface. Add the marinated chicken and stir-fry for 5 to 6 minutes or until the chicken is cooked through and browned.
4. Push the chicken to one side of the griddle, then add the sliced red bell pepper and snow peas. Stir-fry the vegetables for 2 to 3 minutes.
5. Whisk the peanut butter and coconut milk in a small bowl until you reach a smooth consistency. Pour this peanut sauce over the chicken and vegetables on the griddle. Toss to combine.
6. Turn off the heat and stir in the lime juice. Season with extra soy sauce or fish sauce.
7. Serve with a side of cooked jasmine rice, topped with chopped roasted peanuts and cilantro.

CHEESY UDON NOODLES

Serving: 2
Prep time: 5 mins
Cooking time: 10 mins

INGREDIENTS:

- 2 packs of udon noodles
- 2 teaspoons of all-purpose flour
- ½ cup of whole milk
- 1 teaspoon of sesame oil
- 2 tablespoons of butter
- ½ teaspoon of chili flakes
- ⅓ cup of shredded mozzarella cheese

- ½ cup of grated Parmesan cheese
- 2 green onions, sliced
- ½ teaspoon of gochugaru (this is Korean chili powder)
- 1 tablespoon of gochujang (this is a spicy Korean paste)

DIRECTIONS:

1. Fill a big pot with water. Use a stovetop or the hot surface of your griddle to boil the water.
2. As the water boils, add the udon noodles. Let them cook for 1 minute so that they get soft. Then, use a strainer to drain the noodles and put them in a bowl.
3. Add the sesame oil to the noodles and mix. Set the noodles aside for now.
4. If you used your griddle to boil the noodles, no need to preheat it. If you used a stovetop, go ahead and preheat your gas griddle on medium heat. Add the butter, and let it melt.
5. When the butter is almost melted, add the all-purpose flour. Use a whisk to stir it very well. Then, add the chili flakes and the whole milk. Keep whisking until you have a roux. A roux is a thick and creamy sauce that is part flour and part fat (butter).
6. Turn the heat down to low. Add the gochujang, the Parmesan cheese, and half of the mozzarella cheese. Stir until the cheese completely melts and the sauce is very cheesy.
7. Add the cooked udon noodles to the cheesy sauce. Follow with the remaining mozzarella cheese. Toss until everything is well mixed.
8. Transfer your cheesy udon noodles to a serving bowl. Sprinkle the sliced green onions and the gochugaru on top.

MEXICAN ELOTE SHRIMP FRIED RICE

Serving: 2
Prep time: 10 mins
Cooking time: 20 mins

INGREDIENTS:

- 1 cup of cooked jasmine rice
- 12 ounces of peeled, deveined shrimp
- 2 ears of fresh corn, shucked
- 2 tablespoons of olive oil
- 4 tablespoons of crumbled cotija cheese
- 2 teaspoons of chili-lime seasoning blend
- 2 tablespoons of chopped fresh cilantro

DIRECTIONS:

1. As always, preheat your griddle to medium-high. Place the shucked ears of corn directly on the hot surface and rotate it until you see charred spots. This should take 8 to 10 minutes. Remove the grilled corn and set it aside to cool.

2. In the same griddle space, pour in the olive oil. Once the oil is sizzling, add the shrimp and sauté for 3 to 4 minutes. It should be opaque and cooked through when you're done. Transfer the sautéed shrimp to a plate, or do step 3 simultaneously with step 2.

3. Use a sharp knife to slice the kernels off the grilled corn cob onto the griddle. Sauté the corn kernels for 1 to 2 minutes to heat it through.

4. Add the jasmine rice to the griddle. Toss the rice with the corn kernels so it will toast a little. Do this for no more than 2 to 3 minutes.

5. Return the cooked shrimp to the rice and corn mixture and mix everything with your spatula.

6. Turn off the heat and stir in the cotija cheese and the chili-lime seasoning blend. Toss until the rice is properly coated.

7. Transfer the fried rice to a serving bowl and garnish with cilantro.

TEX-MEX CUISINE

Mexican cuisine has its roots going back centuries to the Mayan and Aztec civilizations. Those cultures laid the foundation for the ingredients and preparation methods defining traditional Mexican food—corn tortillas, beans, chili peppers, and seafood. When Mexican meals made their way up to the Texas border region, they started to take on a new identity. The Texan residents were more than happy to embrace the intense flavors of Mexican food, but not long after, they began putting their own spin on the recipes using the ingredients they had readily available, like beef and flour.

The Mexican restaurants in Texas adapted and started modifying traditional recipes to cater more to local tastes. They'd add extra spices, use more beef, and add melted cheese—things that aren't really found in authentic Mexican cooking. This new style of Americanized Mexican food became known as "Tex-Mex." Luckily, Tex-Mex is griddle-friendly, so you can easily recreate all the signature flavors and textures right at home on your flat top.

TIPS FOR MAKING TEX-MEX ON A GAS GRIDDLE

- Cumin, chili powder, garlic powder, and oregano are the building blocks of Tex-Mex flavor.
- Use the zones on your gas griddle to your advantage.
- Make your own refried beans from scratch for a depth of flavor you can't get from canned versions.
- Tex-Mex revolves around indulgence, so don't worry about getting messy.
- Slice your proteins and vegetables into thin strips so they cook quickly and uniformly.
- Use the griddle's large surface area to cook multiple components of your Tex-Mex meal at the same time.
- Line your griddle with foil or parchment paper before cooking to catch any drips or spills. This might cause uneven heating, however.

KITCHEN TOOLS NEEDED

- Mixing bowl
- Cutting board
- Basting brush
- Serving plates

TEX-MEX FAJITAS

Serving: 6
Prep time: 8 hrs 20 mins
Cooking time: 20 mins

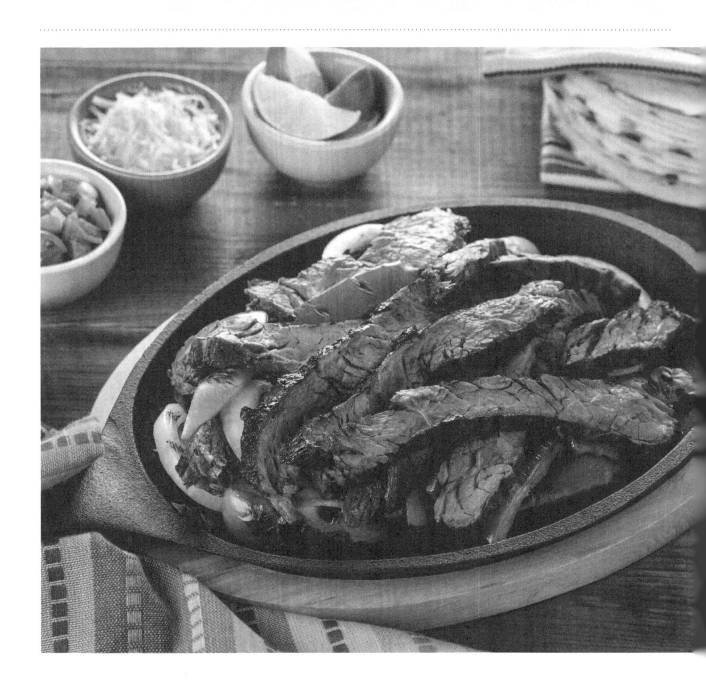

INGREDIENTS:

- ¼ cup of Italian dressing
- ¼ cup of apple cider vinegar
- ¼ cup of low-sodium soy sauce
- 2 tablespoons of Worcestershire sauce
- 2 tablespoons of brown sugar
- 1 tablespoon of lime juice
- 1 crushed garlic clove

For the Fajitas:

- 1 lb. skirt steak, trimmed
- ½ onion, sliced
- ½ green bell pepper, sliced
- 6 flour tortillas

DIRECTIONS:

1. Pour all the marinade ingredients into a shallow bowl. Add the skirt steak and turn it to coat both sides. Cover and let it marinate in the refrigerator for 6 to 8 hours or overnight.
2. Preheat your griddle on medium-high heat.
3. Remove the steak from the marinade and place it on the hot griddle. Cook for 4 to 6 minutes per side or until it is cooked to your liking. Transfer the steak to a cutting board and let it rest for 5 minutes.
4. On the same griddle, add the sliced onion and bell pepper. Cook until the vegetables are soft and sort of burnt. This should take 5 to 7 minutes.
5. Slice the steak against the grain into thin, ¼-inch thick strips.
6. Warm the tortillas on the outer edges of the griddle for 2 to 3 minutes.
7. Serve the steak, onions, and bell peppers with the warm tortillas.

CARNITAS TACO BOWLS

Serving: 2
Prep time: 20 mins
Cooking time: 20 mins

INGREDIENTS:

For the Carnitas:

- 1 lb. boneless pork shoulder, cut into 2-inch cubes
- 1 tablespoon of olive oil
- 1 teaspoon of ground cumin
- 1 teaspoon of dried oregano
- 1 teaspoon of chili powder
- 1 teaspoon of salt
- ½ teaspoon of black pepper

For the Taco Bowls:

- 1 cup of cooked white rice
- 1 (15 oz) can of black beans, drained and rinsed
- 1 cup of shredded lettuce
- ½ cup of diced tomatoes
- ¼ cup of diced red onion
- ¼ cup of shredded cheddar cheese
- 2 tablespoons of chopped fresh cilantro
- Lime wedges for serving

DIRECTIONS:

1. Mix the pork cubes, olive oil, cumin, oregano, chili powder, salt, and black pepper in a bowl. Mix it well to coat the pork.
2. Preheat your griddle over medium-high heat.
3. Place the seasoned pork cubes on the hot griddle and cook until the pork is browned and cooked through. This takes roughly 12 to 15 minutes.
4. Remove the cooked pork from the griddle and place it on a cutting board. Use two forks to shred the pork into smaller pieces.
5. Warm the cooked white rice on the same griddle for 2 to 3 minutes.
6. Scoop the warm rice into two serving bowls.
7. Top the rice with the shredded carnitas, black beans, lettuce, tomatoes, red onion, cheddar cheese, and cilantro.
8. Serve the taco bowls with lime wedges on the side.

BEEF TINGA TOSTADAS

Serving: 4
Prep time: 15 mins
Cooking time: 30 mins

INGREDIENTS:

For the beef tinga:

- 1 lb. beef, diced
- 1 tablespoon of olive oil
- 1 medium onion, diced
- 3 minced garlic cloves
- 1 chipotle chili in adobo sauce, minced
- 1 (14.5 oz) can of diced tomatoes
- 1 teaspoon of cumin
- 1 teaspoon of oregano
- ½ teaspoon of salt
- ¼ teaspoon of black pepper

For the Tostadas:

- 4 corn tortillas
- 1 tablespoon of olive oil

For the Toppings:

- 1 cup of shredded lettuce
- ½ cup of diced tomatoes
- ¼ cup of crumbled queso fresco
- 2 tablespoons of chopped cilantro
- 1 lime, cut into wedges

DIRECTIONS:

1. Mix the beef, olive oil, cumin, oregano, salt, and black pepper in a large bowl. Make sure to coat the beef on all sides.
2. Preheat your griddle on medium-high heat.
3. Place the beef chunks on the hot griddle and cook for 8 to 10 minutes. The beef should be cooked through and browned. Transfer the cooked beef to a plate.
4. Add the diced onion to that same spot and sauté for 5 minutes. Add the minced garlic and chipotle chili, and cook for 1 or 2 more minutes.
5. Add the diced tomatoes (with their juices) to the griddle, along with the cooked beef. Stir to combine, and leave the mixture to simmer for 5 to 7 minutes so the sauce can thicken.
6. While the beef tinga is simmering, brush both sides of the corn tortillas with the remaining 1 tablespoon of olive oil. Place the tortillas on the griddle and cook both sides for 2 to 3 minutes each. You want to get it crispy and golden brown.
7. Place the crispy tostadas on plates and top with the beef tinga mixture, shredded lettuce, diced tomatoes, crumbled queso fresco, and chopped cilantro.
8. Serve with a side of lime wedges.

CHICKEN BURRITOS

Serving: 4
Prep time: 10 mins
Cooking time: 20 mins

INGREDIENTS:

- 2 boneless, skinless chicken breasts (about 1 lb. total)
- 1 tablespoon of chili powder
- 1 teaspoon of cumin
- 1 teaspoon of garlic powder
- ½ teaspoon of onion powder
- Salt and pepper for seasoning
- 4 large flour tortillas
- 1 cup of shredded cheddar or Mexican blend cheese
- ½ cup of cooked black beans
- ½ cup of diced tomatoes
- ¼ cup of diced onion
- Salsa, sour cream, and guacamole for serving (optional)

DIRECTIONS:

1. Season the chicken breasts on both sides with chili powder, cumin, garlic powder, onion powder, salt, and pepper.
2. Preheat your griddle to medium-high. Place the seasoned chicken breasts on the hot griddle and cook both sides for 5 to 6 minutes. Ensure the chicken is cooked and no longer pink in the center.
3. Remove the cooked chicken from the griddle and let it rest for 5 minutes, then shred or chop it into bite-sized pieces. Or just move it to a cooler spot on your griddle and shred it there.
4. Return the shredded chicken to the hot griddle and cook for 2 to 3 more minutes. Stir it until it is heated through.
5. Place the flour tortillas on the griddle and warm them for about 1 minute on each side until they are soft and pliable.
6. Assemble the burritos by placing some of the shredded chicken, black beans, diced tomatoes, onion, and shredded cheese down the center of each tortilla.
7. Fold the bottom of the tortilla over the filling, then fold in the sides and continue rolling up into a burrito shape.
8. Place the assembled burritos seam-side down on the griddle and cook for 3 minutes.
9. Serve the chicken burritos warm, with salsa, sour cream, and guacamole on the side if you want.

MEDITERRANEAN CUISINE

Mediterranean cuisine is the traditional cooking styles and ingredients found in the countries surrounding the Mediterranean Sea. This cuisine is diverse and largely influenced by the region's geography, climate, and cultural histories. You'll find the Greek, Italian, Spanish, French, and Middle Eastern populations encircling the Mediterranean Sea.

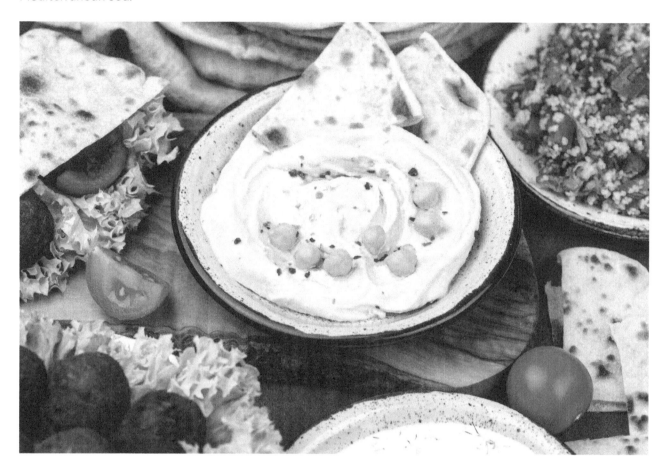

These people have been perfecting this style of cooking for centuries, each area imprinting it with its own exclusive character. Coastal regions, for instance, are known for their abundant seafood, while inland areas rely more on meat, dairy, and produce from the land. This means paella in Spain and moussaka in Greece.

Some common ingredients in Mediterranean cuisine include olive oil, grains, beans, vegetables, cheese, and wine. The main recipes often feature pasta, rice, bread, and different meats and fish—all things that can be maneuvered on a gas griddle to produce the most satisfying meals.

TIPS FOR MAKING MEDITERRANEAN FOOD ON A GAS GRIDDLE

- Marinades, spices, and fresh herbs will give you bold and bright flavors.
- Finish dishes with a pour of premium olive oil or nut oils.
- Don't be afraid of powerful, pungent flavors from ingredients like garlic, olives, and capers.
- Roasted potatoes can be paired with almost everything.

- Wooden skewers
- Mixing bowls
- Food processor
- Cutting board
- Salad bowl

SOUVLAKI

Serving: 2
Prep time: 2 hrs 10 mins
Cooking time: 12 mins

INGREDIENTS:

For the Kabobs:

- 2 tablespoons of olive oil
- 1 clove of garlic, minced
- 1 tablespoon of lemon juice
- ½ teaspoon of dried oregano
- ¼ teaspoon of salt
- 12 ounces of skinless, boneless chicken breast chopped into bite-sized pieces
- 2 wooden skewers, soaked in water for 15 minutes

For the Sauce:

- ⅓ cup of plain Greek yogurt
- ¼ cucumber, peeled, seeded, and grated
- 1 teaspoon of olive oil
- 1 teaspoon of white vinegar
- ½ clove of garlic, minced
- Pinch of salt

DIRECTIONS:

1. Mix the olive oil, 1 clove of garlic, lemon juice, oregano, and ¼ teaspoon of salt in a medium bowl. Add the chicken pieces and mix to coat. Cover this and put it in the fridge to marinate for 2 hours.
2. In the meantime, make the tzatziki sauce. Get a smaller bowl, mix the Greek yogurt, grated cucumber, olive oil, white vinegar, ½ clove of garlic, and a pinch of salt. Cover it and refrigerate for 1 or 2 hours so the flavors blend.
3. Preheat your gas griddle to medium-high.
4. Thread the marinated chicken pieces onto the soaked wooden skewers.
5. Place the chicken skewers on the hot griddle. Cook for 5 to 6 minutes per side. Turn it occasionally until the chicken is cooked through and a little scorched.
6. Serve the souvlaki hot, with the tzatziki sauce on the side.

FALAFEL

Serving: 2
Prep time: 15 mins
Cooking time: 15 mins

INGREDIENTS:

- ½ cup of uncooked chickpeas, soaked for 24 hours, drained, rinsed, and patted dry
- ¼ cup of chopped shallot or yellow onion
- 1½ minced garlic cloves
- ½ teaspoon of lemon zest
- ½ teaspoon of ground cumin
- ½ teaspoon of ground coriander
- ½ teaspoon of sea salt
- ¼ teaspoon of cayenne pepper
- ¼ teaspoon of baking powder
- ½ cup of chopped fresh cilantro leaves and stems, patted dry
- ½ cup of chopped fresh parsley leaves and stems, patted dry
- 1½ teaspoon of extra-virgin olive oil, plus more for drizzling

For Serving:
- 2 pita breads
- ¼ cup of hummus
- ½ cup of diced vegetables (tomato, cucumber)
- 2 tablespoons of chopped fresh herbs (parsley, mint)
- 2 tablespoons of pickled red onions
- 2 tablespoons of Tahini Sauce

DIRECTIONS:

1. Throw the soaked and drained chickpeas, shallot, garlic, lemon zest, cumin, coriander, salt, cayenne, baking powder, cilantro, parsley, and olive oil into a food processor. Pulse until it looks properly mixed but not necessarily pureed.
2. Preheat your griddle to medium-high.
3. Using a 1-tablespoon scoop, form the falafel mixture into thick patties, being careful not to pack them too tightly.
4. Lightly drizzle the falafel patties with olive oil on both sides.
5. Cook the patties on the griddle for 3 to 4 minutes on each side until they look golden brown and crispy on the outside.
6. Warm the pita breads on the griddle for 1 to 2 minutes each side.
7. Spread a layer of hummus inside each pita. Top with the falafel patties, diced vegetables, chopped herbs, pickled onions, and a drizzle of tahini sauce.

CHICKEN SALAD WITH YOGURT DRESSING

Serving: 2
Prep time: 10 mins
Cooking time: 15 mins

INGREDIENTS:

For the Dressing:

- 4 tablespoons of Greek yogurt
- 2 tablespoons of lemon juice
- ½ teaspoon of dried oregano
- ½ teaspoon of dried mint
- 2 tablespoons of extra virgin olive oil

For the Salad:

- 2 boneless, skinless chicken breasts
- 2 cups of spring mix lettuce
- 1 medium tomato, cut into wedges

- 1 English cucumber, sliced
- 1 avocado, pitted and sliced
- 1 small onion, sliced
- ½ cup of kalamata olives
- 3 tablespoons of olive oil
- 1 teaspoon of salt
- 1 teaspoon of pepper
- 3 tablespoons of marinated artichoke hearts
- 3 tablespoons of roasted red pepper strips
- 3 tablespoons of crumbled feta cheese

DIRECTIONS:

1. Preheat your gas griddle to medium-high.
2. Season the chicken breast with olive oil, salt, and pepper.
3. Place the seasoned chicken on the griddle and cook for 5 to 6 minutes on both sides or until it is cooked through. Move it to a cutting board and slice it into bite-sized pieces.
4. To make the dressing, mix the Greek yogurt, lemon juice, dried oregano, dried mint, and olive oil. Adjust the consistency with more lemon juice or oil if you need to.
5. Get a salad bowl and add the spring mix lettuce. Top with the grilled chicken bits, tomato wedges, cucumber slices, avocado slices, red onion, kalamata olives, marinated artichoke hearts, roasted red pepper strips, and crumbled feta cheese.
6. Pour the yogurt dressing over the top of the salad and serve. Eat it on its own or as a side to any dish you prefer. The lentil and quinoa burger on pg. 59 is already perfect for this.

ARMENIAN LOSH KEBAB

Serving: 2
Prep time: 10 mins
Cooking time: 20 mins

INGREDIENTS:

- 4 ounces of ground lamb
- 4 ounces of ground beef
- 1 egg, lightly beaten
- 4 tablespoons of chopped parsley
- 1 teaspoon of cumin

- 1 tablespoons of tomato sauce
- 1 teaspoon of lemon juice
- 1 teaspoon of extra virgin olive oil
- Salt and pepper for seasoning
- ½ diced white onion, divided

DIRECTIONS:

1. Mix the ground lamb, beef, egg, 2 tablespoons of parsley, half of the diced onion, cumin, tomato sauce, lemon juice, olive oil, and a pinch of salt and pepper in a bowl. Mix well to distribute the ingredients as evenly as you can.
2. Shape the mixture into 1 or 2 patties, depending on the size.
3. Preheat your gas griddle over medium-high heat.
4. Carefully place the losh kebab patty onto the hot griddle. Cook each side for four to five minutes or until it is cooked to your liking.
5. Add the remaining diced onion and 2 tablespoons of chopped parsley in another bowl.
6. Once the losh kebab is cooked, transfer it to a plate and garnish with the onion-parsley mixture.
7. Serve the losh kebab warm, either on its own or wrapped in pita bread.

Chapter 8:
Pizza and Flatbreads

PIZZA

Everyone loves pizza one way or another, but wouldn't you like to know how it all began? The origin of pizza is linked to ancient Greece and Rome, where people would put toppings on flatbreads, but the modern pizza you know and love today took off in Naples, Italy, in the 1700s or 1800s. That's where they started making the thin, chewy Neapolitan-style pizzas with simple tomato and mozzarella toppings.

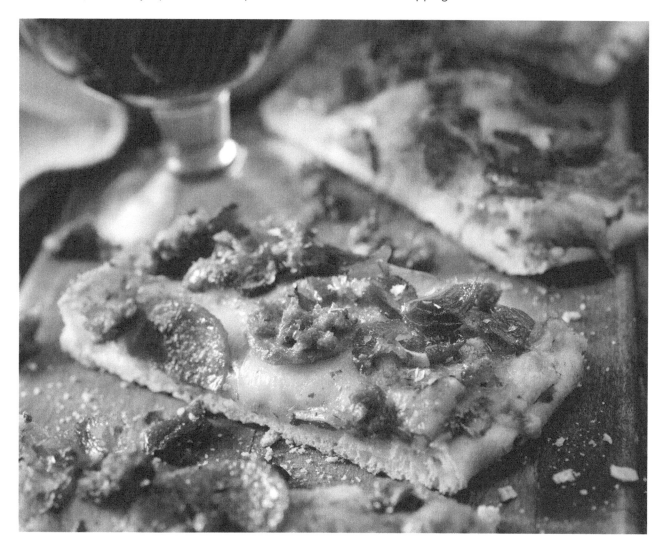

Pizza spread from Italy to other parts of the world, particularly the United States, in the late 19th and early 20th centuries as Italian immigrants brought their food with them. It quickly became a popular fast food in the US, with the development of pizza chains and the introduction of new styles, such as the thick, cheese-laden Chicago deep-dish pizza. Today, everyone loves pizza, regardless of the many regional and national variations. It is one meal that transcends borders, backgrounds, ages, and kitchen equipment. You may not have an oven, but nobody said you can't use your griddle.

TIPS FOR MAKING PIZZA ON A GAS GRIDDLE

- Wipe off any excess oil or butter; you don't want a greasy pizza.
- Aim for a thin, even thickness, around ¼ inch when shaping the pizza dough.
- Use a pizza peel or spatula to lift and check the underside while it cooks.

- Arrange the toppings so the heat can reach the entire surface.
- Dust your pizza peel with flour or cornmeal to prevent it from sticking.
- After the pizza is cooked, brush the edges with a mixture of melted butter and minced garlic for extra flavor.

KITCHEN TOOLS NEEDED

- Mixing bowls
- Rolling pin
- Basting brush
- Cutting board
- Melting dome
- Paper liners

HOMEMADE PIZZA DOUGH

Serving: 2
Prep time: 2 hrs 15 mins
Cooking time: 0 mins

INGREDIENTS:

- 3 cups of bread flour or all-purpose flour
- 1 teaspoon of salt
- 1 teaspoon of instant yeast or active dry yeast
- 1¼ cups of warm water (100-110°F/38-43°C)
- 1 tablespoon of olive oil (optional)

DIRECTIONS:

1. Pour the flour, salt, and yeast into a big bowl. Give that a quick stir to mix it all together.
2. Add the warm water and olive oil (if you're using it). Stir until the dough looks shaggy.
3. Turn that dough out onto a floured surface and get kneading. You'll want to knead it for about 10 minutes until the dough is smooth, elastic, and sort of sticky.
4. Once the dough is ready, place it in an oiled bowl, cover it, and let it rise at room temperature for 1 to 2 hours. You'll know it's ready when it's doubled in size.
5. After the rise, punch down the dough to release any air bubbles. You can use it right away or stick it in the fridge for up to 5 days.
6. When you're ready to make your pizza, just divide the dough into portions and shape or stretch them into your desired crusts.

MARGHERITA PIZZA

Serving: 1 pizza
Prep time: 15 mins
Cooking time: 10 mins

INGREDIENTS:

- 1 lb. pizza dough at room temperature
- 1 cup of shredded mozzarella cheese
- 8 to 10 fresh basil leaves
- 1 cup of canned crushed tomatoes or marinara sauce
- 2 tablespoons of olive oil
- 1 minced garlic clove
- Salt and pepper for seasoning

DIRECTIONS:

1. Preheat your griddle to medium-high.
2. Use your hands or a rolling pin to stretch and shape the pizza dough into a round circle, about ¼ inch thick on a flour-dusted surface.
3. Brush the top of the dough all over with 1 tablespoon of olive oil.
4. Carefully transfer the dough, oiled side down, onto the hot griddle. Cook for 2 to 3 minutes until the bottom is toasted.
5. Flip the dough over and brush the other side with the remaining tablespoon of olive oil.
6. Spread the crushed tomatoes or marinara sauce evenly over the dough, leaving a ½-inch border.
7. Sprinkle the shredded mozzarella cheese over the sauce.
8. Tear or chiffonade (thinly slice) the fresh basil leaves and scatter them on top.
9. Sprinkle a pinch of salt and pepper.
10. Cover the griddle or use a melting dome and cook for 3 or 5 more minutes, until the cheese is melted and the crust is crispy on the bottom.
11. Slide the cooked pizza off the griddle and onto a cutting board. Slice and serve.

MEAT LOVERS PIZZA

Serving: 1 pizza
Prep time: 10 mins
Cooking time: 12 mins

INGREDIENTS:

- 1 lb. pizza dough at room temperature
- 1 cup of tomato sauce or BBQ sauce
- 2 cups of shredded mozzarella cheese
- ½ cup of sliced pepperoni

- ½ lb. Italian sausage, casing removed
- ½ lb. ground beef
- 2 tablespoons of olive oil
- Salt and pepper for seasoning

DIRECTIONS:

1. Get your toppings ready. Cook the Italian sausage and ground beef on the griddle over medium-high heat until they brown and crumble. Drain any excess fat.
2. Dust a flat, clean surface with flour, and use your hands to stretch and shape the pizza dough into a circle.
3. Brush the top of the dough with 1 tablespoon of olive oil.
4. Place the oiled dough on the hot griddle. Cook for 2 to 3 minutes to toast it.
5. Flip the dough over and brush the other side with the remaining tablespoon of olive oil.
6. Spread the sauce evenly over the dough, leaving a ½-inch border.
7. Sprinkle the shredded mozzarella cheese all over the sauce.
8. Top with the sliced pepperoni, crumbled Italian sausage, and crumbled ground beef.
9. Season with salt and pepper.
10. Cover the griddle or use a melting dome and cook for 3 more minutes to melt the cheese and crisp the underside.
11. Slide the cooked pizza off the griddle and onto a cutting board. Slice and serve.

MUSHROOM AND ONION PIZZA

Serving: 1 pizza
Prep time: 15 mins
Cooking time: 30 mins

INGREDIENTS:

- 1 lb. pizza dough at room temperature
- 1 cup of marinara sauce
- 2 cups of shredded mozzarella cheese
- 8 ounces of sliced portobello mushrooms

- 1 large onion, thinly sliced
- 2 tablespoons of olive oil, divided
- Salt and pepper for seasoning

DIRECTIONS:

1. Preheat your griddle over medium-high heat.
2. Add 1 tablespoon of the olive oil to the hot griddle. Follow with the sliced mushrooms and cook for 5 to 7 minutes, stirring until the mushrooms are brown and soft. Remove the mushrooms to a plate or to a cooler spot on the griddle.
3. Pour the remaining tablespoon of olive oil onto the griddle surface. Add the thinly sliced onions and cook for 10 or 12 minutes, stirring until the onions are caramelized and golden brown. Move the onions to the place with the mushrooms.
4. Dust a flat surface with flour. Use your hands or a rolling pin to stretch and shape the pizza dough into a circle.
5. Glaze the top of the dough with a light coating of olive oil.
6. Place the dough, oiled side down, on the hot griddle. Cook for 2 to 3 minutes.
7. Flip the dough over and spread the marinara sauce over the crisp surface.
8. Sprinkle the mozzarella cheese on top of the sauce.
9. Top the pizza with the sautéed mushrooms, caramelized onions, and a sprinkle of salt and pepper.
10. Cover with a melting dome and cook for 3 to 5 minutes to melt the cheese and toast the bottom.
11. Transfer the pizza to a cutting board. Slice into triangles and serve.

PINEAPPLE AND BACON PIZZA

Serving: 1 pizza
Prep time: 10 mins
Cooking time: 25 mins

INGREDIENTS:

- 3 ounces of bacon, sliced into 1-inch pieces
- 1 can of pineapple chunks in juice, drained and halved
- 1 tablespoon of brown sugar

- 1 lb. pizza dough
- ½ cup of BBQ sauce
- 4 ounces of shredded Monterey Jack cheese
- 2 green onions, sliced

DIRECTIONS:

1. Heat the gas griddle on medium. Add the sliced bacon pieces and cook for 5 minutes until they are crispy and brown on the edges. Move it to a paper towel-lined plate, and drain most of the bacon grease from the griddle.
2. Add the drained and halved pineapple chunks to the griddle along with the brown sugar. Sauté and stir for 5 minutes until the pineapple is caramelized and sticky on the edges. Remove it from the heat.
3. Stretch or roll the pizza crust into a circle and oil one side with olive oil. Place the oiled side directly on the hot griddle to toast for 2 or 3 minutes until the crust is light brown.
4. Flip the crust over and spread the BBQ sauce over the surface, leaving a tiny border untouched. Sprinkle the shredded Monterey Jack cheese on top.
5. Top the pizza with the cooked bacon pieces and the caramelized pineapple chunks.
6. Cover the pizza with a melting dome and cook for 8 or 10 more minutes to melt the cheese and toast the bottom.
7. Slide it off the griddle, top it with the green onions, slice it into 8 pieces, and serve.

CHICAGO-INSPIRED THIN-CRUST PIZZA

Serving: 1 pizza
Prep time: 2 hrs 15 mins
Cooking time: 10 mins

INGREDIENTS:

- ¼ cup of lukewarm water
- 1 teaspoon of sugar
- ½ teaspoon of active dry yeast
- 1 tablespoon of unsalted butter, melted and cooled
- ¾ cup of all-purpose flour
- 2 tablespoons of yellow cornmeal
- ¼ teaspoon of salt
- 1 tablespoon of unsalted butter, room temperature

- 2 tablespoons of tomato sauce
- 2 ounces of thinly sliced pepperoni
- ½ cup of shredded mozzarella and provolone cheese blend
- ½ teaspoon of dried oregano
- ¼ teaspoon of red pepper flakes (optional)
- Additional toppings (e.g., sliced mushrooms, diced bell peppers, sliced Italian sausage, chicken bits)

DIRECTIONS:

1. Add the lukewarm water, sugar, and yeast to a small bowl. Give it about 10 minutes to get foamy. Stir in the melted butter.
2. In a bigger bowl, mix the flour, cornmeal, and salt. Pour in the yeast mixture and stir until a dough forms.
3. Flour your work surface and knead the dough for 2 to 3 minutes until soft.
4. Shape it into a ball, put it in a greased bowl, cover it, and let it rise for 2 hours or until it doubles in size.
5. After the dough has risen, punch it down and roll it into a very thin, round shape.
6. Preheat your griddle over medium-high heat. Spread that room-temperature butter all over one side of the dough.
7. Place the dough, butter-side down, on the hot griddle. Cook it for 3 or 4 minutes.
8. Flip it and top the browned side with the tomato sauce, pepperoni, shredded cheese, oregano, and red pepper flakes (if you're into that). Add any other toppings you'd like.
9. Cover the pizza with a melting dome and cook it for another 2 or 3 minutes to melt the cheese.
10. Slice and serve.

Flatbreads are simple, versatile, and found in cultures all across the globe. These thin, flat discs of dough have been feeding people for thousands of years, and they're still going strong today. Some of the most well-known examples of flatbreads include:

- **Pita:** A Middle Eastern bread that puffs up when baked, creating a pocket that is usually stuffed with ingredients.
- **Naan:** A leavened, tandoor-baked South Asian flatbread, often flavored with garlic or other seasonings.
- **Chapati/Roti:** Unleavened wheat flatbreads from the Indian subcontinent cooked on a griddle.
- **Tortilla:** A thin, circular flatbread made from masa (nixtamalized corn flour) that originates in Mexico.
Lavash: A paper-thin Armenian flatbread that can be baked, grilled, or cooked on a griddle.
- **Focaccia:** An Italian flatbread that is baked in the oven, often topped with herbs, vegetables, or cheese.
- **Injera:** A spongy, fermented Ethiopian flatbread made from teff flour.

Flatbreads are portable, keep well, and are part of cherished cultural traditions and social rituals. Despite being thin, simple discs of dough, they can do it all. They are great for scooping, wrapping, and plain eating, making an amazing base for many toppings. You can make your own flatbreads at home with just a few basic ingredients and your gas griddle.

TIPS FOR MAKING FLATBREADS ON A GAS GRIDDLE

- While your flatbreads cook, use a pastry brush to baste the tops with flavored oils like garlic-infused olive oil or spiced sesame oil.
- Make extra dough and portion it into balls. Freeze the raw dough balls on a baking sheet, then transfer them to a freezer bag. This way, you can bake fresh flatbreads anytime.
- If you don't have a baking sheet, use just a light coating of oil on the griddle. Too much oil will cause the dough to become greasy and soggy.
- Instead of your hands, use a bench scraper or dough cutter to transfer the shaped dough rounds to the hot griddle.
- Grate frozen butter into the dry ingredients before mixing the dough. The frozen butter will create lovely pockets in the flatbread as it melts.

KITCHEN TOOLS NEEDED

- Mixing bowls
- Clean towel
- Baking sheet
- Plastic wrap
- Basting brush
- Melting dome
- Rolling pin
- Airtight container or Ziplock bag
- Wire rack

YOGURT FLATBREAD

Serving: 6
Prep time: 1 hrs 15 mins
Cooking time: 5 mins

INGREDIENTS:

- 1½ teaspoons of honey
- 1 package of active dry yeast (2¼ teaspoons)
- 2¼ cups of all-purpose flour, plus extra for dusting
- ½ teaspoon of kosher salt
- ⅓ cup of plain yogurt
- Vegetable oil for the griddle

DIRECTIONS:

1. Mix 2 tablespoons of warm water with the honey in a small bowl until the honey dissolves. Stir in the yeast and let it sit for 5 minutes until it bubbles.

2. While you wait, mix the flour and salt in a separate bowl. Make a well in the center and add the yogurt and ⅓ cup of warm water. Stir the water and yogurt together in the well, then stir in the yeast mixture. Using a spatula, fold the mixture together until it forms a rough ball of dough.

3. Lightly dust a clean work surface with flour and knead the dough for 3 to 5 minutes until it becomes smooth. When the dough begins to stick to your hands, dust them with flour and continue kneading.

4. Cover the dough with a clean towel and leave it to rise for 1 hour or until it doubles in size.

5. Punch down the dough and divide it into six equal pieces, about 3½ ounces each. Roll each piece into a ball, then use your hands to flatten and stretch each ball into a roughly 6-inch round.

6. Heat your griddle on medium-high and grease the surface with vegetable oil.

7. Cook the flatbreads in batches, placing them on the hot griddle. Cook for 1 or 2 minutes until bubbles appear on the top and the bottom is cooked and deep brown in spots. Flip and cook the other side for another 1 to 2 minutes.

8. Place the cooked flatbreads on a baking sheet to cool.

9. Serve with Greek salad on top.

RAMAZAN PIDESI

Serving: 4
Prep time: 40 mins
Cooking time: 18 mins

INGREDIENTS:

- ½ cup of warm milk
- 2 tablespoons of olive oil
- 1½ teaspoons of granulated sugar
- 1½ teaspoons of instant dry yeast
- ½ teaspoon of kosher salt
- 1 large egg, white and yolk separated

- 2¼ cups of all-purpose flour, plus extra for dusting
- 1½ tablespoons of yogurt
- 1 tablespoon of toasted white sesame seeds
- 1 tablespoon of nigella seeds (Also called black cumin, roman coriander or black seed. They are small black pungent seeds)

DIRECTIONS:

1. Stir the warm milk, ½ cup of warm water, and olive oil in a large bowl. Add the sugar, yeast, salt, and egg whites. Stir again.
2. Using a strong spoon, stir in the flour, 1 cup at a time, ending with the ¼ cup. The dough will be sticky now.
3. Cover the bowl with plastic wrap and a kitchen towel. Place it in a room temperature spot to rise for 30 minutes until it almost doubles in size.
4. Remove the covering and transfer the dough to a well-floured surface. Sprinkle the dough with about ½ tablespoon flour and fold the edges inward with your hands.
5. Flip the dough so the sealed part is on the bottom, then dust the top of the dough with a little flour and shape it into a ball.
6. Heat your griddle over medium-high heat, and line it with a baking sheet.
7. Make the glaze. Mix the egg yolk, yogurt, and 1½ teaspoons of water in a small bowl.
8. Gently press the dough down a bit with your fingers. Spread the glaze over the top of the dough and, using your fingers, spread the dough into an oval shape ½-inch thick.
9. Using your fingers again, make indentations in a full circle 1 inch from the edge of the dough. Then, make indentations inside the circle across the dough in lines 1 inch apart. Repeat the process in the opposite direction to create a diamond or square pattern.
10. Apply more glaze over the dough and follow with a sprinkle of sesame and nigella seeds.
11. Carefully lift the dough and place it on the hot griddle. Cover it with a melting dome and cook for 18 minutes until it is golden on top.
12. Take it off the griddle and cover it loosely with a kitchen towel for 10 minutes before serving.

HOMEMADE TORTILLAS

Serving: 12
Prep time: 1 hrs 10 mins
Cooking time: 25 mins

INGREDIENTS:

- 2 cups of all-purpose flour
- ¾ teaspoon of kosher salt
- ¾ teaspoon of baking powder
- ¼ cup of extra virgin olive oil or other neutral oil
- ¾ cup of warm water

DIRECTIONS:

1. Mix the flour, salt, and baking powder in a bowl.
2. Add the oil and warm water to the dry ingredients. Use a strong spoon or your hands to mix it until a shaggy dough forms.
3. Turn the dough out onto a floured surface and knead for 2 minutes until it is smooth and elastic.
4. Divide the dough into 12 equal pieces. Roll each piece into a smooth ball and let it sit for 30 minutes to an hour.
5. Heat your griddle on medium and spray a light coat of oil over the surface.
6. Working one dough ball at a time, use a rolling pin to roll it out into a round tortilla shape as flat as you can go. Try to keep the thickness even.
7. Place the rolled-out tortilla on the hot griddle. Cook for 40 seconds to 1 minute, or until the bottom has a few pale brown spots and the top is bubbly.
8. Flip the tortilla and cook the other side for 15-20 seconds or until golden.
9. Repeat the rolling and cooking with the remaining dough balls.
10. Use the warm tortillas immediately for the quesadillas starting at pg. 45, or let them cool completely before storing.
11. Store your tortillas in an airtight container or Ziplock bag at room temperature for up to 24 hours or in the refrigerator for up to 1 week.

PITA BREAD

Serving: 6
Prep time: 2 hrs 30 mins
Cooking time: 35 mins

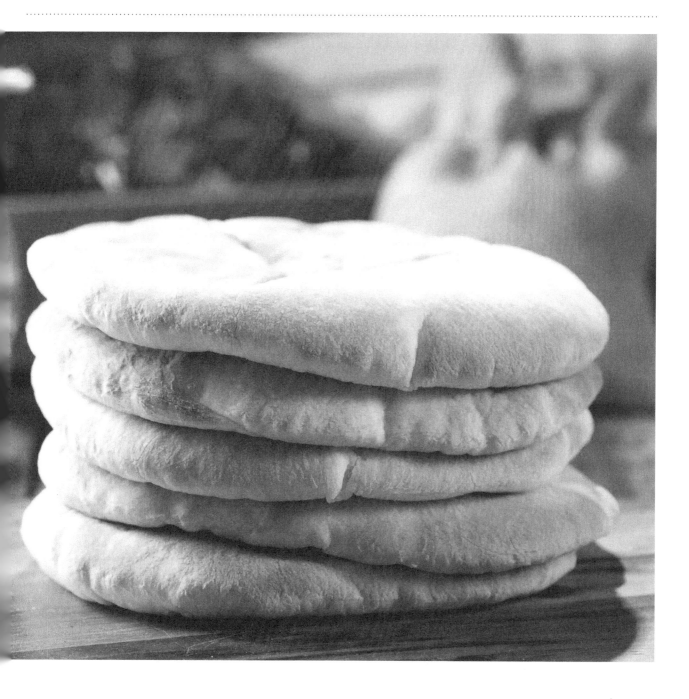

INGREDIENTS:

- 1 package (2¼ teaspoons) of active dry yeast
- 1 teaspoon plus ½ tablespoon of sugar
- 2¼ cups of bread flour, plus more for dusting
- ¾ teaspoon of sea salt
- 1½ tablespoons of extra-virgin olive oil, plus more for the bowl
- ½ cup of whole-milk Greek yogurt
- ½ cup of warm water

DIRECTIONS:

1. Activate the yeast by mixing warm water, yeast, and 1 teaspoon of sugar in a bowl. Let the mixture sit for 5 minutes until it's frothy on top.
2. Mix the bread flour, salt, and remaining ½ tablespoon of sugar in a large mixing bowl. Add the yeast mixture, 1½ tablespoons of olive oil, and yogurt, and mix until you get a shaggy dough.
3. Turn the dough onto a flour-dusted surface and knead for 7 to 10 minutes until the dough is soft and a little sticky. Use a little more flour if needed.
4. Place the dough in an oiled bowl, cover it with a towel or plastic wrap, and let it rise for almost 2 hours until it doubles in size.
5. Punch down the dough and divide it into six equal pieces. Cover them and let them rise for another 20 minutes.
6. Heat your griddle on medium-high and line it with parchment paper.
7. Working with one piece of dough at a time, use your hands or a rolling pin to stretch and flatten it into a thin round shape.
8. Place the pita dough on the hot griddle. Cook for 2 to 3 minutes per side or until the pita is puffed up and brown.
9. Transfer the cooked pitas to a wire rack to cool. Repeat with the remaining dough pieces.
10. Serve the pitas warm or at room temperature, with your favorite dipping sauce on the side. They will keep in an airtight container at room temperature for up to 3 days.

Chapter 9:
Quick and Easy Weeknight Meals

Gas Griddle Cookbook

Master Easy and Flavorful Recipes
to Elevate Your Grilling and Wow Every Time

There are those days when the thought of slaving away in the kitchen for hours on end for just one meal is enough to make a shiver run down your spine. However, with the right tools and a little know-how, you can prepare yummy, homemade meals easily, even on your busiest evenings.

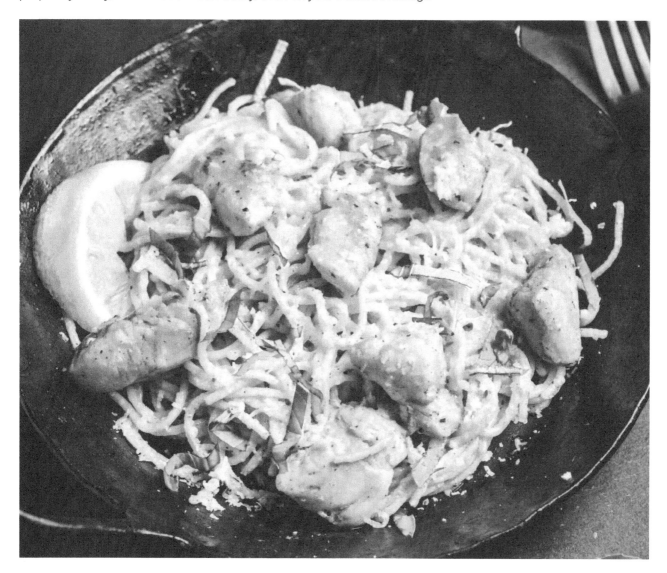

A griddle is THE secret to preparing quick, easy meals requiring minimal effort and cleanup. You might wonder what exactly qualifies as a "quick and easy" meal in this context. You're looking at recipes that take 30 minutes or less from start to finish, use just a handful of basic, affordable ingredients, and involve little to no prep work other than a bit of chopping or mixing. No elaborate, time-consuming recipes here—just simple, delicious meals that you can get on the table in a matter of moments. The following recipes are a few good examples.

TIPS FOR MAKING QUICK AND EASY WEEKNIGHT MEALS ON A GAS GRIDDLE

- Items like tortillas, eggs, sliced cheese, and pre-chopped vegetables make for easy, customizable meals.
- Chop onions, grate cheese, or cook ground meat ahead of time so you can throw everything together when it's meal time.
- Cook multiple elements of a meal simultaneously to save time.

- A few go-to spice blends or sauces can make basic ingredients taste amazing.
- Use a light hand when greasing the griddle—you generally won't need much oil or butter.
- Try the "cook once, eat twice" method by making extra portions for lunches or freezing.
- Have a few "no-fail" go-to recipes on hand for those ultra-busy weeknights.

KITCHEN TOOLS NEEDED

- Mixing bowls
- Paper towels
- Basting brush
- Metal spatula
- Metal pot
- Stovetop
- Saucepan
- Cooking spray
- Potato masher
- Serving plates

BACON AND EGG FRIED RICE

Serving: 4
Prep time: 10 mins
Cooking time: 15 mins

INGREDIENTS:

- 4 large eggs
- ½ teaspoon of kosher salt
- 4 ounces of bacon
- 1 medium yellow onion
- 2 teaspoons of vegetable oil

- 3 cups of cooked rice
- ¼ teaspoon of ground black pepper
- ½ teaspoon of sugar
- 2 tablespoons of soy sauce
- 2 tablespoons of chopped green onion

DIRECTIONS:

1. Cut the bacon into tiny pieces and finely dice the onion.
2. Heat the vegetable oil on the griddle over medium heat.
3. Crack the eggs into a small bowl, season with a pinch of salt, and beat well.
4. Pour the beaten eggs onto the hot griddle and gently scramble them. When they are almost cooked through, move them to a bowl or another spot on the griddle.
5. Pour the bacon pieces onto the griddle and cook until they are crisp and the fat has rendered. Place the bacon with the scrambled eggs.
6. Add the diced onion to the griddle and stir-fry until they are translucent.
7. Add the cooked rice to the translucent onions and stir-fry for 2 to 5 minutes until the rice is starting to crisp. Use a spatula to break up any clumps.
8. Season the rice with black pepper, then add the sugar and soy sauce. Stir for another minute or so until the rice is steaming and warmed through.
9. Stir in the bacon and scrambled eggs.
10. Garnish the rice with the green onions, and serve warm with sausages on the side.

SCALLOPS AND CAPER SAUCE

Serving: 4
Prep time: 5 mins
Cooking time: 10 mins

INGREDIENTS:

- 8 large sea scallops
- Kosher salt for seasoning
- Ground black pepper for seasoning
- 4 tablespoons of unsalted butter, divided
- 1 tablespoon of olive oil

- 2 shallots, minced
- 2 minced cloves of garlic
- 3 tablespoons of capers, drained and rinsed
- ½ cup of white wine

DIRECTIONS:

1. Season both sides of the scallops with salt and pepper.
2. Preheat your griddle over high heat. Melt 1 tablespoon of the butter and the olive oil on the griddle.
3. When the butter has melted, add the scallops and sear, flipping once halfway through, until they are golden brown on both sides and nearly opaque all the way through. This should take 3 or 4 minutes total.
4. Transfer the scallops to a plate and turn the griddle knob to medium heat.
5. Melt another 1 tablespoon of butter on the griddle. Add the minced shallot and garlic and cook. Stir for 2 minutes until they are soft and light brown.
6. Stir in the capers and cook for 1 minute or until fragrant.
7. Pour the white wine into the mix and cook. Stir for about 3 minutes or until the liquid reduces by a little.
8. Turn off the heat and melt the remaining butter into the sauce. Season the sauce with salt and pepper.
9. Spoon the caper-wine sauce over the seared scallops and serve over roasted garlic Alfredo (Pg. 80).

GLAZED SALMON

Serving: 2
Prep time: 7 mins
Cooking time: 15 mins

INGREDIENTS:

- 1 tablespoon of brown sugar
- ½ tablespoon of Dijon mustard
- ½ tablespoon of honey
- ½ teaspoon of kosher salt

- ¼ teaspoon of ground black pepper
- ¼ teaspoon of red pepper flakes
- 2 (8-ounce) skin-on salmon filets

DIRECTIONS:

1. Grab a small bowl and mix the brown sugar, Dijon mustard, honey, salt, black pepper, and red pepper flakes until it's smooth, like a glaze.

2. Pat the filets dry, especially on the skin side if you plan on eating it.

3. Preheat your griddle to medium-high and drizzle some cooking oil on the surface.

4. Place the salmon filets on the griddle skin-side down. Let them cook for 5 to 7 minutes until the skin gets crispy.

5. Flip the filets over and slather the glaze over the tops. Use the back of a spoon or a basting brush to get it everywhere.

6. Let the salmon keep cooking for another 5 minutes or more. You'll know it's done when it flakes easily with a fork and the internal temperature reaches 125°F to 130°F.

7. Transfer the glazed salmon filets to your serving plate or serve over a bed of coconut rice.

MASALA FISH STICKS

Serving: 4
Prep time: 15 mins
Cooking time: 25 mins

INGREDIENTS:

- 1 pound of cod fish filets
- 1 teaspoon of kosher salt, divided
- ¼ cup of all-purpose flour
- 1 teaspoon of garam masala
- ½ teaspoon of cayenne pepper
- Black pepper and salt for seasoning
- 1 large egg
- ⅓ cup of whole milk
- ¾ cup of panko breadcrumbs
- Cooking spray

DIRECTIONS:

1. Pat the fish filets dry with paper towels. Cut them into finger-length pieces that are about ¾ inch wide. Sprinkle the fish sticks with ½ teaspoon of salt.

2. Mix the flour, garam masala, cayenne pepper, and a pinch of salt and black pepper in a shallow bowl.

3. Beat the egg and milk in a separate bowl, then sprinkle in the remaining ½ teaspoon of salt.

4. Place the panko breadcrumbs, a small amount of salt, and pepper in a third bowl.

5. Preheat your griddle to medium-high and coat the surface with cooking spray.

6. Starting with one fillet at a time, coat each fillet in the flour mixture, then dip it in the egg wash, letting any excess drip off. Finally, dip it in the panko breadcrumbs and press gently to help the crumbs stick.

7. Place the breaded fish sticks on the hot griddle a few inches apart. Cook for 3 or 4 minutes per side or until they're golden brown and crispy.

8. Serve your fish sticks warm with your choice of dipping sauce on the side.

CHOPPED CHEESE

Serving: 4
Prep time: 5 mins
Cooking time: 15 mins

INGREDIENTS:

- 1½ lb. ground beef
- 1 white onion, chopped
- 3 cloves of garlic, chopped
- ¾ teaspoon of kosher salt
- ¼ teaspoon of black pepper
- 2 teaspoons of Worcestershire sauce

- 4 hoagie or bolillo rolls, sliced almost all the way through
- 8 slices of American cheese
- 4 tablespoons of mayonnaise
- Shredded iceberg lettuce for serving
- Tomato slices for serving

DIRECTIONS:

1. Preheat a griddle on low.
2. Add the ground beef to the griddle and cook, stirring to break it up as it cooks, until it is browned and most of the fat has gone out. This may take only 5 or 6 minutes.
3. Turn the heat up to medium, add the onions and garlic, and cook for another 3 to 4 minutes until the vegetables have softened.
4. Season the beef mixture with salt, pepper, and Worcestershire sauce. Take it off the heat.
5. Toast the rolls on the griddle over medium heat for 1 or 2 minutes per side.
6. Scoop a quarter of the beef mixture and place it on the griddle. Top the beef with 2 slices of American cheese.
7. Use a metal spatula to chop the cheese roughly into the beef mixture to melt.
8. Spread 1 tablespoon of mayonnaise on one side of a toasted roll, then place the roll, mayo side down, on top of the chopped beef and cheese mix.
9. After 30 seconds, use a spatula to flip the roll, keeping the filling inside. If any filling falls out, just use the spatula to add it back to the roll.
10. Add shredded lettuce and tomato slices to the sandwich.
11. Cut each sandwich in half and serve.

PARMESAN LEMON CHICKEN

Serving: 2
Prep time: 15 mins
Cooking time: 15 mins

INGREDIENTS:

- 2 chicken cutlets
- Kosher salt and ground black pepper for seasoning
- 3 tablespoons of all-purpose flour
- 3½ tablespoons of grated Parmesan, divided
- 1 tablespoon of unsalted butter
- 1 teaspoon of vegetable oil

- 2 minced cloves of garlic
- ½ cup of chicken stock
- 2 tablespoons of dry white wine
- ½ tablespoon of freshly squeezed lemon juice
- 1 tablespoon of heavy cream
- 1 tablespoon of chopped parsley leaves

DIRECTIONS:

1. Season the chicken cutlets with salt and a little bit of pepper.
2. Get a shallow bowl and mix some flour and Parmesan cheese.
3. Take each chicken cutlet and coat it with the Parmesan mixture.
4. Heat some butter and vegetable oil on your griddle set to medium heat.
5. When the griddle is hot, add the chicken and cook each side for 4 or 5 minutes until golden brown and cooked through. Transfer them to a plate.
6. Lower the heat to medium-low and sprinkle some flour over the drippings. Whisk this until it looks somewhat brown, which should take roughly a minute.
7. Gradually whisk in some chicken stock, white wine, and lemon juice. Let that simmer for 3 minutes until the sauce thickens.
8. Stir in some Parmesan, heavy cream, and parsley. Season the sauce with salt and pepper.
9. Return the cooked chicken to the griddle and let it cook in the sauce for 2 or 3 minutes, spooning the sauce over the chicken.
10. Serve on its own or with roasted vegetables.

SHRIMP TACOS

Serving: 4
Prep time: 10 mins
Cooking time: 10 mins

INGREDIENTS:

- 2 minced cloves of garlic
- 1½ teaspoons of freshly squeezed lime juice
- 1 teaspoon of chili powder
- 1 tablespoon of unsalted butter, melted
- ½ teaspoon of smoked paprika
- Salt and black pepper for seasoning
- ½ teaspoon of ground cumin
- 1 lb. medium shrimp, peeled and deveined

- 1½ tablespoons of chopped fresh cilantro leaves
- Sliced avocado
- 4 or 6 small flour or corn tortillas
- Sliced jalapeños
- Shredded cabbage
- Hot sauce
- Crumbled queso fresco

DIRECTIONS:

1. Preheat your griddle to medium-high and spray with a light coat of cooking oil.
2. Mix the melted butter, garlic, lime juice, chili powder, paprika, cumin, ½ teaspoon salt, and ¼ teaspoon pepper in a small bowl.
3. Place the shrimp in the bowl and coat them in the mix.
4. Arrange the seasoned shrimp on the hot griddle in a single layer. Cook both sides for 2 to 3 minutes until the shrimp are pink and cooked through.
5. Move the cooked shrimp to a cooler spot on the griddle and stir in the chopped cilantro.
6. Warm the tortillas on both sides on the griddle for 30 to 60 seconds.
7. Place some of the shrimp in the center of each tortilla. Follow with shredded cabbage, sliced avocado, sliced jalapeños, and crumbled queso fresco.
8. Serve your tacos immediately, with hot sauce on the side for those who want a little extra heat.

CHICKEN STIR-FRY MEATBALLS

Serving: 2
Prep time: 10 mins
Cooking time: 10 mins

INGREDIENTS:

For the Meatballs:

- Cooking spray
- ½ lb. ground chicken
- 2 tablespoons of chopped scallions, plus more for garnish
- 1 large egg, beaten
- 2 tablespoons of plain breadcrumbs
- 1 teaspoon of finely chopped garlic
- 1 teaspoon of toasted sesame oil
- 1½ teaspoons of low-sodium soy sauce
- Black pepper

For the Sauce:

- 1 teaspoon of cornstarch
- 2 tablespoons of chicken stock
- 1 tablespoon of low-sodium soy sauce
- 1 teaspoon of chopped garlic
- 1 teaspoon of chopped ginger
- 1½ teaspoons of unseasoned rice vinegar
- 1 tablespoon of honey
- ½ teaspoon of toasted sesame oil
- Cooked rice for serving
- Toasted sesame seeds, for garnish

DIRECTIONS:

1. Spray some cooking spray on your griddle surface and preheat it to medium-high.
2. Mix the ground chicken, chopped scallions, beaten egg, breadcrumbs, garlic, sesame oil, and soy sauce in a bowl. Add a pinch of black pepper and mix it again.
3. Shape the chicken mixture into 5 or 6 meatballs.
4. Place the meatballs on the heated griddle and cook the sides for 4 to 5 minutes until they're brown and fully cooked.
5. While the meatballs are cooking, prepare the sauce. Into a small bowl, pour the cornstarch and 1 teaspoon of water. Stir until you get a consistent mixture.
6. Place a small saucepan on an unused area of your griddle surface. Add the cornstarch mixture, chicken stock, soy sauce, garlic, ginger, rice vinegar, honey, and sesame oil into it. Cook over medium-low heat, whisking constantly, for 1 or 2 minutes. The result will be a thick sauce.
7. Once the meatballs are done, remove them from the griddle and add them to the sauce. Toss to coat.
8. Serve your stir-fried meatballs with cooked rice and garnish with some extra chopped scallions and toasted sesame seeds.

PASTA CARBONARA

Serving: 2
Prep time: 10 mins
Cooking time: 20 mins

INGREDIENTS:

- 2 slices of chopped bacon
- 1 large egg, plus 3 large egg yolks
- ¾ ounces of grated Parmesan (about 2 tablespoons)
- ¾ ounces of pecorino, grated (about 2 tablespoons)
- Salt and black pepper for seasoning
- 4 ounces of spaghetti

DIRECTIONS:

1. Preheat your griddle over medium heat. Add the chopped bacon and cook for 6 or 8 minutes until crisp and browned. Transfer the cooked bacon to a paper towel-lined plate, reserving about 2 tablespoons of the bacon fat in the griddle.
2. Get a bowl and whisk the whole egg and egg yolks. Stir in the grated Parmesan, pecorino, and 1 tablespoon of the reserved bacon fat. Sprinkle as much black pepper as you want.
3. Boil the spaghetti in a pot of salted water over the griddle or a stovetop. Drain the pasta and save ¼ cup of the cooking water.
4. Very slowly, while whisking constantly, pour 2 tablespoons of the hot pasta cooking water into the egg mixture to temper the eggs.
5. Add the drained spaghetti to the griddle and coat it with the remaining bacon fat. Pour the egg mixture over the hot pasta and toss quickly to mix, letting the eggs gently cook and create a creamy sauce.
6. If the sauce seems too thick, pour a splash more of the pasta water to thin it out.
7. Take it off the heat and stir in the cooked bacon pieces. Sprinkle with salt and pepper, and serve.

CHINESE ORANGE CHICKEN

Serving: 4
Prep time: 10 mins
Cooking time: 15 mins

INGREDIENTS:

For the Sauce:

- Zest from ½ an orange, plus ¼ cup of fresh orange juice
- 1½ teaspoons of soy sauce
- 1½ teaspoons of packed brown sugar
- 1½ teaspoons of white vinegar
- 1 tablespoon of chicken stock
- ½ teaspoon of freshly grated ginger
- ½ teaspoon of cornstarch

For the Chicken:

- 1½ tablespoons of cornstarch
- 2 large egg whites
- 1 lb. boneless, skinless chicken thighs, diced into 1-inch bits
- ½ cup of all-purpose flour
- ¼ teaspoon of baking powder
- Salt and black pepper
- 1½ or 2 cups of canola oil
- Sliced scallions for garnish
- Cooked rice for serving

DIRECTIONS:

1. Use a small bowl to whisk the orange zest and juice, soy sauce, brown sugar, vinegar, chicken stock, and ginger. Stir in ½ teaspoon of cornstarch and keep it for later.
2. Whisk 1 tablespoon of cornstarch and the egg whites in another bowl until it looks frothy. Add the chicken pieces and let them sit for 5 minutes.
3. Mix the flour, baking powder, and remaining ½ tablespoon of cornstarch. Season that with a pinch of salt and pepper.
4. Remove the chicken bits from the egg white mixture one by one and coat them in the flour mixture. Shake off any excess.
5. Heat the canola oil on your griddle set to medium-high.
6. Fry the chicken in batches for 3 to 4 minutes each side until it looks golden brown and cooked. Move the fried chicken to a paper towel-lined plate.
7. Lower the heat to medium-low. Add the prepared orange sauce and cook for 2 or 3 minutes until it thickens.
8. Add the fried chicken to the sauce and gently toss to coat.
9. Serve immediately over cooked rice, garnished with sliced scallions.

TEX-MEX CHICKEN MEATBALLS

Serving: 2
Prep time: 8 mins
Cooking time: 5 mins

INGREDIENTS:

- ½ lb. ground chicken
- 1 large egg, beaten
- Cooking spray
- 2 tablespoons of plain breadcrumbs
- 1 teaspoon of chopped garlic
- 2 tablespoons of chopped onion
- 2 tablespoons of chopped hatch chiles

- ¼ teaspoon of ground cumin
- Salt and black pepper for seasoning
- ¼ teaspoon of chili powder
- 1 cup of roughly chopped romaine lettuce
- Guacamole, salsa, and grated cheese for serving

DIRECTIONS:

1. Preheat your griddle to medium-high and coat the surface with cooking spray.
2. Thoroughly mix the ground chicken, beaten egg, breadcrumbs, onion, garlic, hatch chiles, chili powder, cumin, and a pinch each of salt and pepper in a bowl.
3. Divide the chicken mixture into 5 to 6 equal-sized meatballs.
4. Place the meatballs on the preheated griddle and cook all sides for 5 minutes or until they are browned and cooked through.
5. Arrange the chopped romaine lettuce on two serving plates.
6. Top the lettuce with the cooked meatballs.
7. Serve with toppings like guacamole, salsa, and grated cheese.

STEAK AND MASHED POTATOES

Serving: 2
Prep time: 10 mins
Cooking time: 30 mins

INGREDIENTS:

- 12 ounces of Yukon gold potatoes, peeled and diced into chunks
- Salt and black pepper
- ½ cup of fresh or frozen peas
- 1 teaspoon of lemon zest plus 1 tablespoon of lemon juice
- 2 tablespoons of olive oil, divided
- 2 strip steaks
- 1 small shallot, thinly sliced
- ¼ cup of dry white wine
- 1 tablespoon of unsalted butter

DIRECTIONS:

1. Boil some salted water in a saucepan on the griddle. Pour in the potato chunks and let them cook for 15 to 18 minutes until they are soft enough to mash. Add the peas for the last 3 minutes. Drain everything and put them back in the pan.
2. Mix in lemon zest, lemon juice, and a tablespoon of olive oil. Mash everything until it looks smooth and creamy. Sprinkle salt and pepper over the mashed potatoes and mix again. Keep the potatoes warm on the griddle while you cook the steak.
3. Heat 1 tablespoon of olive oil on the griddle over medium-high heat. Season both sides of the steaks with salt and pepper.
4. Cook both sides for 3 to 5 minutes each for medium-rare doneness. Move them to a tray and let them cool.
5. Lower the heat to medium-low and add the sliced shallots to the griddle. Cook these for around 2 to 4 minutes until they're soft.
6. Pour the white wine into the shallots, scraping up any browned bits from the bottom. Let the wine boil until it is reduced by half.
7. Turn off the heat and stir in the butter until it melts.
8. Slice the steak against the grain. Serve it drizzled with the shallot-wine sauce alongside the mashed potatoes.

Chapter 10:
Entertaining with Your Griddle

Hosting friends and family is one of life's great joys, isn't it? But it is also quite stressful, especially when you have to feed a crowd.

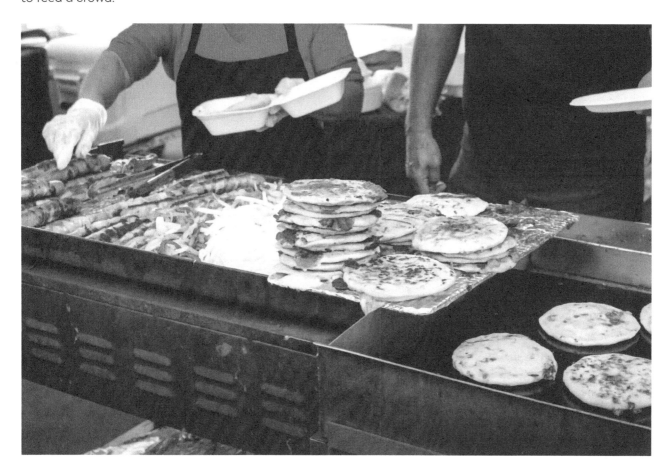

Instead of staying chained to the stove, anxiously watching the clock, you can be out there catching up, drink in hand, while your griddle does what it does best. Thanks to the one kitchen equipment that does it all, you'll be the host(ess) with the most(est).

Beyond the practical benefits, cooking on a griddle adds an interactive, communal element to your events, depending on what you're cooking. You can bet that guests will love the option of customizing their foods, be it topping their pancakes with their preferred fruits and drizzles or assembling their own burgers just the way they like them. There will be conversation and laughter as everyone gets involved in cooking. No one has to feel left out, and you don't have to be a short-order cook juggling multiple meals. The griddle does the work for you, freeing you up to enjoy quality time with your guests. Isn't that the whole point of having people over?

TIPS FOR SERVING AND HOSTING GUESTS WITH A GAS GRIDDLE

- Timing: You don't want your guests to be left waiting around, hungry, while you're still cooking. Try to have everything timed properly so the food comes off the griddle hot and ready to serve all at once. That way, you can just bring it straight to the table.
- Arrangement: Pretend you're an artist arranging a still-life painting. Think about how you can make the food look visually appealing on the plate. Mix colors, textures, and shapes so it's interesting to the eye. You want it to look like it belongs in a fancy restaurant, not just thrown together.

- Garnishes: A little goes a long way when it comes to garnishes. Just a sprinkling of fresh herbs, a squeeze of lemon, or a few onion strings can elevate the dish's look and make it feel special.
- Sauces and condiments: Set out some tasty dipping sauces, spreads, or spicy condiments on the side. That way, people can customize their bites and try different flavor combinations.
- Temperature: No one likes lukewarm food. Keep everything hot by transferring it straight from the griddle to heated serving dishes. You can even use a warming tray or chafing dish to maintain that just-cooked temperature.
- Mise en place: Do as much prep work as you can ahead of time. Get all your plates, utensils, and garnishes ready to go. That way, when it's time to serve, you can focus on making it look great instead of scrambling to find what you need.
- Family-style serving: For a more laid-back, communal vibe, arrange the dishes on big platters or boards that people can pass around and help themselves. This makes way for conversation and lets your guests customize their own plates exactly how they want.
- Portion control: When you're dishing individual servings, try not to go overboard. You want your guests to feel satisfied, not completely stuffed. Stick to reasonable 4 to 6-ounce portions of the main proteins and leave room for all the sides and accouterments.
- Encourage conversation: Set up the griddle and serving areas in a way that encourages mingling and chatting. You want people to feel comfortable getting up, grabbing refills, and talking with each other in between courses.
- Serve in courses: Instead of just piling everything on the table at once, try serving the meal in stages. Start your guests off with a little appetizer straight off the griddle, then bring out the main dishes after they've had a chance to relax and chat for a bit. It keeps things interesting and gives you more control over the pacing.

Kitchen Tools Needed
- Mixing bowls
- Saucepan
- Basting brush
- Big platter
- Muffin tins
- Cutting board
- Wooden skewers
- Aluminum foil
- Pitcher
- Ziplock bags
- Food processor
- Toothpicks
- Microwave
- Serving plates

SRIRACHA WINGS

Serving: 6
Prep time: 2 hrs 10 mins
Cooking time: 20 mins

INGREDIENTS:

- 6 chicken wings, with skins
- 1 teaspoon of ground coriander
- 1½ teaspoons of canola oil
- ¼ teaspoon of pepper
- ¼ teaspoon of garlic salt

Sauce:

- ¼ cup of orange juice
- 1 tablespoon of lime juice
- 2 tablespoons of unsalted butter, cubed
- 2½ tablespoons of sriracha chili sauce
- 2 tablespoons of chopped fresh cilantro
- 1½ tablespoons of honey

DIRECTIONS:

1. Mix the chicken wings, canola oil, ground coriander, garlic salt, and pepper in a bowl. Toss to coat the wings. Cover and refrigerate for 2 hours or up to overnight.
2. Heat your griddle over medium heat. Arrange the chicken wings in a single layer and cook for 15 to 18 minutes, turning every so often.
3. Meanwhile, prepare the sauce. In a small saucepan set on your flat top, melt the butter. Whisk in the orange juice, sriracha, honey, and lime juice.
4. During the last 5 minutes of cooking the wings, baste them with some of the Sriracha sauce.
5. Transfer the wings to a large bowl. Pour in the remaining Sriracha sauce and coat the wings as much as you can.
6. Sprinkle the chopped cilantro over the sauced wings and serve immediately.

BURGER BAR

Serving: 12
Prep time: 30 mins
Cooking time: 45 mins

INGREDIENTS:

- 2 lbs. ground beef
- 1 teaspoon of salt
- ½ teaspoon of black pepper
- ½ teaspoon of garlic powder
- 12 soft burger buns or brioche rolls split in half

Toppings:

- Sliced cheddar or American cheese
- Sliced tomatoes
- Lettuce leaves
- Sliced onions
- Pickles
- Bacon, cooked
- Sautéed mushrooms
- Caramelized onions
- Sliced avocado
- Chipotle aioli or other condiments

DIRECTIONS:

1. Mix the ground beef, salt, pepper, and garlic powder in a big bowl. Mix gently to combine the ingredients.
2. Shape the beef into 12 fairly even patties, about 4 or 5 inches wide and half an inch thick.
3. Preheat your flat top to medium-high. Cook those burger patties for 3 or 4 minutes per side until they're cooked through.
4. While the burgers are sizzling, toast the buns on the griddle until they're golden brown.
5. Get a big platter or smaller bowls and arrange all the fillings on display.
6. Once the burgers are done, transfer them to a serving platter.
7. Let your guests go on to build their dream burgers. Make arrangements for some plates and extra napkins too. The griddle will keep the patties warm while everyone gets creative.

STUFFED PORTOBELLO MUSHROOMS

Serving: 4
Prep time: 5 mins
Cooking time: 15 mins

INGREDIENTS:

- 4 large Portobello mushroom caps, stems removed
- 2 tablespoons of olive oil, plus more for brushing
- ½ cup of panko breadcrumbs
- ½ cup of grated Parmesan cheese

- ¼ cup of cream cheese, softened
- 2 minced cloves of garlic
- 1 teaspoon of dried oregano
- ¼ teaspoon of red pepper flakes (optional)
- ¼ teaspoon of salt
- A pinch of black pepper

DIRECTIONS:

1. Preheat your griddle on medium-high heat.
2. Mix the panko, Parmesan, cream cheese, garlic, oregano, red pepper flakes (if using), salt, and pepper in a medium-sized bowl.
3. Brush the portobello caps all over with olive oil.
4. Place the caps, gill-side up, on the hot griddle. Cook for 3 to 4 minutes until the caps begin to soften.
5. Flip the caps over and cook for another 2 to 3 minutes. This should soften the mushrooms even more.
6. Remove the caps from the griddle and flip them back over so the gill side faces up.
7. Generously stuff each portobello cap with the cheesy panko mixture, pressing it down lightly to compact it.
8. Place the stuffed caps back on the griddle, stuffing-side up. Cook for 4 to 5 minutes or until the stuffing is hot and melty.
9. Carefully transfer the stuffed portobello caps to a serving plate.
10. Serve warm, garnished with extra Parmesan, chopped parsley, or any other toppings you prefer.

GRILLED STEAK AND CAULIFLOWER FLORETS

Serving: 8
Prep time: 30 mins
Cooking time: 20 mins

INGREDIENTS:

For the Cauliflower Florets:

- 20 ounces of cauliflower florets
- Juice of 2 limes
- ½ cup of fresh cilantro, chopped
- ½ cup of fresh dill, chopped
- 2 teaspoons of salt
- 2 teaspoons of dried oregano
- 2 teaspoons of black pepper

For the Steak:

- 3 pounds of skirt steak
- 2 tablespoons of apple cider vinegar
- ¼ cup of olive oil
- 3 teaspoons of salt
- 2 tablespoons of hot sauce
- 1 teaspoon of onion powder
- 1 teaspoon of ground cumin
- 1 teaspoon of smoked paprika
- 1 teaspoon of black pepper

For the Cilantro-Lime Dressing:

- 1 cup of plain Greek yogurt
- Juice of 2 or 3 limes
- 2 teaspoons of olive oil
- 1 large bunch of cilantro
- ½ teaspoon of paprika
- Salt and black pepper for seasoning

For the Peach Salsa:

- 2 peaches or nectarines, chopped and pitted
- 1 cup of cherry tomatoes, quartered
- 1 medium red onion, chopped
- Juice of 4 limes
- ½ cup of fresh cilantro, chopped
- Olive oil (Optional)
- Apple cider vinegar (Optional)
- Salt and black pepper for seasoning

DIRECTIONS:

1. Pour all the peach salsa ingredients into a bowl and mix well. Season it with as much salt and pepper as you like. If you'll be using olive oil and apple cider vinegar, now is the time to add those.

2. Put all the dressing ingredients in a food processor and blend until it is smooth. Set it aside.

3. Cut the skirt steak in half crosswise to make two long pieces. Put all the steak seasoning ingredients into a small bowl and mix. Rub this seasoning mix all over the steak pieces. Let that sit at room temperature for 20 to 30 minutes.

4. While the steak is marinating, work on the cauliflower. Get a large bowl and toss the cauliflower florets with the cilantro, dill, lime juice, salt, pepper, and oregano.

5. Preheat your griddle on high heat and coat with cooking spray.

6. Place the seasoned cauliflower florets directly on the hot griddle. Let them cook for 15 to 20 minutes until the cauliflower is tender.

7. While the cauliflower is cooking, go ahead and place the marinated steak pieces on a different spot on the griddle. Cook for 2 to 3 minutes per side for medium-rare, or a little longer if you want them more well-done.

8. Once the steak is cooked, transfer it to a cutting board and let it rest for 5 minutes before slicing it into strips.

9. Serve the cauliflower florets drizzled with cilantro lime dressing with the sliced steak and peach salsa on the side.

ZUCCHINI FRIES

Serving: 4
Prep time: 15 mins
Cooking time: 15 mins

INGREDIENTS:

- 2 medium zucchinis, sliced into ½-inch thick fry-shaped pieces
- 1 cup of panko breadcrumbs
- ½ cup of grated Parmesan cheese
- 1 tablespoon of garlic powder
- 1 tablespoon of dried basil
- 1 teaspoon of salt
- 1 teaspoon of black pepper

- 2 eggs, beaten

Greek Yogurt Dip:
- 1 cup of plain Greek yogurt
- 1 tablespoon of lemon juice
- 2 tablespoons of chopped fresh chives
- ¼ teaspoon of salt
- ¼ teaspoon of black pepper

DIRECTIONS:

1. Preheat your griddle to medium-high.
2. Mix the panko breadcrumbs, grated Parmesan, garlic powder, dried basil, salt, and pepper in a shallow bowl.
3. Dip the zucchini pieces first into the beaten eggs, then dredge them through the breadcrumb mixture, pressing lightly to help the coating stick.
4. Place the breaded zucchini pieces in a single layer on the griddle. Let them cook for 2 to 3 minutes per side until golden brown and crunchy.
5. Make your sauce while the zucchini fries cook. Mix the Greek yogurt, lemon juice, chopped chives, salt, and pepper in a small bowl.
6. Move the fries to a serving plate. Let your guests serve themselves with a side of dipping sauce.

PIGS IN A BLANKIE

Serving: 18
Prep time: 15 mins
Cooking time: 30 mins

INGREDIENTS:

- 6 hot dogs
- 1 sheet of puff pastry, cut into 6 even rectangles
- 6 slices of cheddar cheese

DIRECTIONS:

1. Preheat your flat top to medium-high.
2. Lay out the puff pastry rectangles, top each one with a slice of cheddar cheese, and follow with a hot dog right on top of the cheese.
3. Gently roll the puff pastry around the hot dog and cheese, creating tiny wrapped bundles.
4. Slice each one into 3 even sections. This should give you 18 bite-sized pieces.
5. Spray a light sheen of cooking oil on the griddle surface and arrange the pastries on it. Leave an inch of space between each one.
6. Cook each side of a piece for 2 to 3 minutes or until the pastry is golden brown and flaky. The cheese should be melted as well.
7. Transfer the pigs in a blankie to a serving plate.

MUSHROOM TOASTS

Serving: 4
Prep time: 10 mins
Cooking time: 25 mins

INGREDIENTS:

- 42 ounces of brown mushrooms, sliced
- 3 tablespoons of olive oil
- 12 slices of bread, 1-inch thick
- 9 minced garlic cloves
- 2 teaspoons of kosher salt
- 9 scallions, thinly sliced
- ¾ cup of heavy cream
- 12 poached eggs
- 2 teaspoons of paprika, plus extra for garnish

DIRECTIONS:

1. Preheat your griddle to medium. Pour olive oil over the surface.
2. Add the garlic and paprika to the griddle and let that sizzle for 1 minute.
3. Stir in the mushrooms and salt, adding a bit more oil if the griddle looks dry. Sauté and stir the mushrooms for 15 to 20 minutes or until they are browned.
4. Stir in the heavy cream and scallions (reserve a few scallions for later). Cook for 2 or 3 minutes to heat the cream.
5. Move the mushroom mixture to another spot on the griddle.
6. Place the bread slices on a clean spot on the griddle and toast them, flipping once, until golden brown on both sides.
7. Scoop the mushroom mix onto the toasted bread slices.
8. Top each toast with a poached egg.
9. Lightly dust the eggs with extra paprika and garnish with the reserved scallions.
10. Serve your mushroom toast immediately.

BALSAMIC GLAZED FIG AND PORK TENDERLOIN SKEWERS

Serving: 12
Prep time: 30 mins
Cooking time: 10 mins

INGREDIENTS:

- 1 or ½ lb. pork tenderloin, trimmed
- ¼ cup of balsamic vinegar
- 3 tablespoons of honey
- ½ cup of crumbled blue cheese
- 2 teaspoons of olive oil
- 12 dried figs, halved
- 1 tablespoon of Dijon mustard
- 12 cherry tomatoes
- 4 basil leaves, thinly sliced

- 1 teaspoon of salt
- 1 tablespoon of smoked paprika
- 1 teaspoon of onion powder
- ½ teaspoon of garlic powder
- 1 teaspoon of pepper
- ¼ teaspoon of cayenne pepper
- ½ teaspoon of white pepper
- Cooked rice, optional

DIRECTIONS:

1. Cut the pork tenderloin into 1-inch chunks.
2. Mix the smoked paprika, salt, pepper, onion powder, garlic powder, white pepper, and cayenne in a small bowl. Rub this mixture all over the pork chunks. Put it in the fridge until you're ready to cook.
3. To make the glaze, get a medium bowl and whisk the balsamic vinegar, honey, Dijon mustard, and olive oil. Keep it for later.
4. Preheat your griddle over medium-high heat.
5. Thread the seasoned pork chunks and fig halves onto water-soaked wooden skewers.
6. Place the skewers on the hot griddle. Cook for 8 to 10 minutes total, turning once in a while, until the pork is fully cooked.
7. Brush the skewers with the balsamic glaze in the last few minutes.
8. Turn off the heat and let the kabobs stand for 5 minutes. Stick a cherry tomato on each skewer.
9. Put the skewers on a serving platter, and sprinkle the pork and figs with crumbled blue cheese and sliced basil leaves.
10. Serve with some cooked rice if you want.

SHRIMP WRAPPED IN BACON

Serving: 18
Prep time: 20 mins
Cooking time: 20 mins

INGREDIENTS:

- ¼ cup of sugar
- ¼ cup of lemon juice
- 2 tablespoons of olive oil
- 3 teaspoons of paprika
- 1 teaspoon of salt
- 1 teaspoon of garlic powder

- 1 teaspoon of black pepper
- 18 uncooked shrimp, peeled and deveined, with tails
- 9 partially cooked bacon strips, halved lengthwise
- Lemon wedges (Optional)

DIRECTIONS:

1. Mix the sugar, lemon juice, olive oil, paprika, salt, garlic powder, and black pepper in a small bowl to make the marinade.
2. Pour a quarter cup of the marinade into a large, shallow dish. Add the shrimp and let them sit for 15 minutes, flipping now and then to coat.
3. Cover and refrigerate the remaining marinade to use for basting later.
4. Preheat your flat top to medium-high.
5. Drain the shrimp from the marinade, discarding the used marinade. Wrap each shrimp with a piece of the halved bacon strips and secure each one with a toothpick.
6. Place the bacon-wrapped shrimp directly on the hot griddle. Cook both sides for 3 or 4 minutes each until the shrimp turn pink.
7. While cooking, baste the shrimp with the reserved marinade.
8. Turn off the heat and serve hot, with lemon wedges on the side.

FLANK STEAK CROSTINI

Serving: 24
Prep time: 10 mins
Cooking time: 40 mins

INGREDIENTS:

- ¾ lb. beef flank steak
- 24 ¼-inch thick baguette slices (1½ baguettes)
- 3 tablespoons of olive oil
- ½ cup of finely chopped fresh portobello mushrooms
- 3 minced garlic cloves

- ¼ cup of shredded part-skim mozzarella cheese
- 1 teaspoon of dried basil
- ¼ teaspoon of salt
- 2 tablespoons of grated Parmesan cheese
- 1 tablespoon of minced chives
- ¼ teaspoon of pepper

DIRECTIONS:

1. Preheat your griddle to medium-high.
2. Sprinkle some salt and pepper on the flank steak.
3. Place the steak on the hot griddle and cook it for 4 to 6 minutes on each side or until it's cooked how you like it.
4. Take the steak off the griddle and let it cool for 5 minutes. Then, cut it into thin slices against the grain.
5. Mix the olive oil, minced garlic, and dried basil in a small bowl. Brush that mix onto the baguette slices.
6. Toast the baguette slices on the griddle for 2 or 3 minutes per side until golden brown.
7. Pile the toasted baguette slices with chopped portobello mushrooms and shredded mozzarella cheese.
8. Put the loaded slices back on the griddle and cook them for 2 or 3 more minutes until the cheese is melted.
9. Take the crostini off the griddle and top each one with a slice of the grilled flank steak, a sprinkle of Parmesan cheese, and a pinch of minced chives.

FAJITA BAR

Serving: 4
Prep time: 1 hr 15 mins
Cooking time: 25 mins

INGREDIENTS:

For the Steak:

- 2 lbs. flank steak or skirt steak cut into thin strips
- 2 tablespoons of olive oil
- 2 teaspoons of chili powder
- 1 teaspoon of cumin
- 1 teaspoon of garlic powder
- 1 teaspoon of onion powder
- 1 teaspoon of salt
- ½ teaspoon of black pepper

For the Vegetables:

- 2 bell peppers, sliced into strips
- 1 red onion, thinly sliced
- 2 tablespoons of olive oil
- 1 teaspoon of salt
- ½ teaspoon of black pepper

Toppings/Accompaniments:

- Flour tortillas or corn tortillas
- Shredded cheddar or Monterey Jack cheese
- Sour cream
- Salsa
- Guacamole
- Diced tomatoes
- Shredded lettuce
- Lime wedges

DIRECTIONS:

1. Mix the steak strips, olive oil, chili powder, cumin, garlic powder, onion powder, salt, and pepper in a big bowl. Toss the steak to coat it with the flavors. Leave it to marinate for 30 minutes to 1 hour.
2. Use another bowl to toss the bell pepper strips and onion slices with some olive oil, salt, and pepper.
3. Preheat your griddle over high heat.
4. Place the steak strips on it and cook both sides for 2 or 3 minutes, until they're cooked through and look a little charred. Move them to a plate.
5. Lower the heat to medium and cook the vegetables for 4 to 6 minutes until they're soft and a bit charred. Scoop them onto a plate.
6. Put all the toppings on the counter or table so everyone can make their own fajitas.

SPICY BUTTERED CORN ON THE COB

Serving: 12
Prep time: 5 mins
Cooking time: 15 mins

INGREDIENTS:

- 12 ears of corn, husks removed
- 3 minced cloves of garlic
- 9 tablespoons of melted butter
- Juice of 6 limes
- 1 cup of sweet chili sauce
- Crushed red pepper flakes (optional)
- 3 tablespoons of sriracha
- Salt and black pepper
- Freshly chopped cilantro, for garnish
- 3 red Thai chilies, sliced, for garnish

DIRECTIONS:

1. Mix the sweet chili sauce, melted butter, sriracha, minced garlic, and lime juice in a bowl. Season this chili-lime butter mixture with salt and pepper. If using, now is the time to add a pinch or two of red pepper flakes.
2. Preheat your griddle over medium-high heat.
3. Place the corn cobs on the griddle. Cook the cobs for 10 to 15 minutes max, turning them occasionally until they are soft and scorched in spots.
4. As the cobs cook, brush them with some of the prepared chili-lime butter mixture.
5. When they are cooked through, transfer them to a serving platter.
6. Drizzle the remaining chili-lime butter over the grilled corn, making sure to coat all the cobs.
7. Garnish the buttered corn with the chopped cilantro and sliced red Thai chilies.
8. Serve hot.

MINI CHEESE SANDWICHES

Serving: 12
Prep time: 5 mins
Cooking time: 10 mins

INGREDIENTS:

- 24 slices of bread
- 12 ounces of cream cheese at room temperature
- 1 cup of chopped sun-dried tomatoes
- 1 teaspoon of black pepper
- 1½ cups of grated parmesan cheese (or cheddar, pepper jack, mozzarella)
- Butter (For the griddle)

DIRECTIONS:

1. Preheat your griddle to medium.
2. Place the bread slices on a chopping board or clean surface, and cut off the crusts with a sharp knife.
3. Mix the cream cheese, sun-dried tomatoes, and black pepper in a bowl until it's smooth enough and thoroughly combined.
4. Spread the creamy filling on half of the bread slices, and then top with the other half to make mini sandwiches.
5. Drop some butter on the griddle and wait for it to melt.
6. Place the mini sandwiches on the griddle and cook for a few minutes on each side until they're golden brown.
7. Flip them and sprinkle some grated parmesan cheese on top.
8. Cook for a few more minutes until the cheese melts, then take them off the griddle to cool before serving.

MEXICAN STREET CORN

Serving: 6
Prep time: 5 mins
Cooking time: 15 mins

INGREDIENTS:

- 2 tablespoons of oil
- 6 cups of frozen corn kernels
- 1 teaspoon of salt
- 1 teaspoon of black pepper
- 2 tablespoons of mayonnaise

- ½ cup of chopped cilantro
- 1 cup of Cotija cheese
- 2 limes, juiced
- 1 teaspoon of Tajin (optional)

DIRECTIONS:

1. Preheat your flat top to medium-high.
2. Coat the entire surface of the griddle with oil.
3. Microwave the corn for 2 to 5 minutes to cook it only partially.
4. Spread the corn out on the preheated griddle. Sprinkle salt and pepper to season it.
5. Cook the corn for 5 to 7 minutes, stirring until it is heated through and a bit scorched.
6. Create a well in the center of the corn and pour the mayonnaise into the center. Fold the corn into the mayonnaise.
7. Squeeze the lime juice over the corn and sprinkle the Cotija cheese on top. Stir to combine.
8. Scoop the corn into a serving dish, garnish with cilantro, and, if you want, sprinkle with Tajin seasoning.

EGG ROLL IN A BOWL

Serving: 6
Prep time: 10 mins
Cooking time: 10 mins

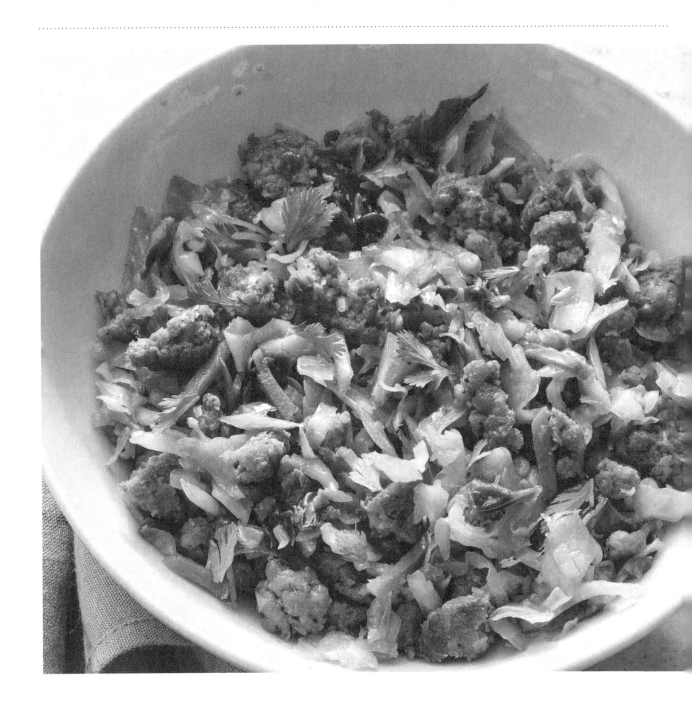

INGREDIENTS:

- 2 tablespoons of vegetable oil
- 3 lbs. ground pork or ground chicken
- 2 onions, diced
- 1 cup of soy sauce
- 3 tablespoons of minced ginger
- 3 tablespoons of minced garlic
- 1 teaspoon of kosher salt
- 3 tablespoons of rice vinegar or lime juice
- 3 (9.5 ounces) Asian salad kits
- 1 teaspoon of black pepper
- ½ cup of sliced green onions
- 1 cup of shredded carrots
- ½ cup of chopped cilantro

Optional Toppings:

- Sesame seeds
- More soy sauce
- Spicy mayo
- Extra green onions
- Yum Yum sauce
- Ginger soy glaze
- Wonton and almond packet from the salad kit
- White or brown rice

DIRECTIONS:

1. Get your griddle preheated on medium.
2. Add the oil to the griddle and use a spatula or basting brush to get it everywhere.
3. Add the onions and ground pork (or chicken) to the griddle. Cook that for 3 to 4 minutes, stirring and flipping it with the spatula so it browns properly.
4. Add the soy sauce, ginger, garlic, vinegar (or lime juice), salt, and pepper. Stir to mix the flavors.
5. Get the Asian salad kits (but leave out the dressing and topping packets for later) and add them to the griddle, along with the carrots, cilantro, and green onions. Cook that for 4 or 5 more minutes, stirring as you go.
6. Scoop the mixture onto a serving platter.
7. Let your guests serve themselves and top their own bowl with their favorite extras, like spicy mayo, ginger soy glaze, sesame seeds, more green onions, soy sauce, yum yum sauce, and don't forget the wonton and almond packet from the salad kit.

BACON-WRAPPED MUSHROOMS

Serving: 18
Prep time: 10 mins
Cooking time: 30 mins

INGREDIENTS:

- 9 partially cooked bacon strips, halved
- 18 fresh portobello mushrooms
- ¾ cup of balsamic vinegar

DIRECTIONS:

1. Get the bacon halves and wrap each mushroom with a piece of it. Use a toothpick to keep it in place.
2. Preheat your griddle over medium-high heat.
3. Put the bacon-wrapped mushrooms directly on the hot griddle.
4. Brush some balsamic vinegar on the mushroom tops.
5. Let them cook for 10 to 15 minutes, flipping them and brushing on more vinegar. Do this until the bacon is crispy and the mushrooms are soft.
6. Keep an eye on them and adjust the heat to make sure the bacon doesn't burn.
7. When they're ready, transfer the bacon-wrapped mushrooms to a serving platter.
8. Serve hot.

SALMON IN FOIL

Serving: 8
Prep time: 30 mins
Cooking time: 20 mins

INGREDIENTS:

- 8 skin-on salmon filets
- Kosher salt and black pepper
- 8 tablespoons of unsalted butter, melted, plus extra for foil
- 4 teaspoons of chopped fresh dill, plus extra for garnish

- 2 teaspoons of chopped garlic
- 2 teaspoons of lemon zest
- 2 red bell peppers, sliced
- 2 cups of corn
- 2 cups of lima beans

DIRECTIONS:

1. Preheat your flat top to medium-high.
2. Sprinkle some salt and pepper on both sides of the salmon filets.
3. Cut 8 large sheets of heavy-duty foil and spread a bit of butter in the middle of each one.
4. Mix the melted butter, 4 teaspoons of chopped dill, garlic, and lemon zest in a small bowl.
5. Put a salmon filet, skin-side down, in the middle of each buttered foil sheet. Pour the butter mixture over each filet.
6. Spread the red bell peppers, corn, and lima beans around the salmon in the foil packets.
7. Wrap the foil tightly around the salmon and vegetables to seal each packet.
8. Place the foil packets on the preheated griddle and cook for 15 to 20 minutes until the salmon is cooked through.
9. Take the packets off the griddle, place them on plates and open the foil.
10. Sprinkle some more fresh dill on the salmon before serving.

BOURBON BBQ PORK CHOPS

Serving: 8
Prep time: 5 mins
Cooking time: 25 mins

INGREDIENTS:

- 1 tablespoon of olive oil
- ¼ teaspoon of cayenne pepper
- 1 cup of ketchup
- 1 tablespoon of chili powder
- ¾ cup of Bourbon
- ¼ cup of cider vinegar
- ¼ cup of molasses

- 2 tablespoons of dark brown sugar
- 1 teaspoon of Worcestershire sauce
- 2 tablespoons of Dijon mustard
- 2 cloves of garlic, pressed
- Kosher salt
- Black pepper
- 8 (1-inch thick) bone-in pork chops

DIRECTIONS:

1. Heat the olive oil and garlic in a medium saucepan over medium heat on the griddle, stirring as you go, until the garlic sizzles but does not brown. This should take 1 minute.
2. Add the chili powder and cayenne pepper. Cook and stir for another minute.
3. Add the ketchup, bourbon, molasses, vinegar, brown sugar, Dijon mustard, and Worcestershire sauce. Let the mixture simmer for 12 to 15 minutes until it thickens. Season with salt and pepper.
4. Season the pork chops generously with kosher salt and black pepper on both sides.
5. Place the seasoned pork chops on a different spot on the griddle. Let it cook, turning once until the internal temperature reaches 135°F. This may take 10 to 14 minutes max.
6. In the last 4 minutes of cooking, baste the pork chops with ⅔ cup of the Bourbon glaze.
7. Move the grilled pork chops to a serving platter and baste them again with the remaining glaze.
8. Serve the pork chops immediately, with any extra glaze on the side for dipping or drizzling.

GRILLED POTATO SALAD WITH BACON VINAIGRETTE

Serving: 10
Prep time: 25 mins
Cooking time: 40 mins

INGREDIENTS:

- 5 lbs. baby Yukon gold potatoes, halved
- 9 tablespoons of olive oil, divided
- ¾ cup of apple cider vinegar
- 9 slices of center-cut bacon, cut into ½-inch pieces
- 3 tablespoons of fresh marjoram, plus extra for garnish

- Black pepper
- 3 cloves of garlic, very finely chopped
- 3 teaspoons of brown sugar
- Kosher salt
- 12 scallions

DIRECTIONS:

1. Preheat your flat top to medium-high.
2. Place the halved potatoes in a large pot and cover with cold salted water. Cover the pot and let the potatoes cook.
3. Reduce the heat to a simmer and cook for 15 to 20 minutes. You'll know it's ready when the potatoes are easily pierced with a knife.
4. Drain the potatoes and let them cool. After that, transfer them to a large bowl and toss with 3 tablespoons of olive oil.
5. Put the bacon in a small saucepan set on one side of the griddle over medium heat. Cook for 5 to 8 minutes or until crisp. Move the bacon to a paper towel-lined plate.
6. Discard all but 1 tablespoon of the bacon drippings from the saucepan. Turn off the heat and pour the vinegar, garlic, and brown sugar into the drippings, scraping up any browned bits.
7. Whisk in the remaining 6 tablespoons of olive oil. Season the vinaigrette with salt and pepper, then transfer it to a bowl.
8. Remove the saucepan and set the griddle to medium heat. Place the potatoes cut-side down on it. Grill them for just 2 or 3 minutes. Grill the scallions too for 4 to 6 minutes. Move the scallions to a cutting board and chop them into pieces.
9. Add the grilled potatoes, chopped scallions, and 3 tablespoons of the fresh marjoram to the bowl with the bacon vinaigrette. Toss to coat, then leave the salad alone for 5 minutes.
10. Sprinkle the crispy bacon over the potato salad and toss again. Season with more salt and pepper.
11. Serve hot, garnished with extra fresh marjoram.

BUTTERMILK BRINED CHICKEN MASALA

Serving: 16
Prep time: 20 mins
Cooking time: 45 mins

INGREDIENTS:

For the Brine:

- 12 cups of buttermilk
- 1 cup of kosher salt
- 8 tablespoons of sugar
- 6 teaspoons of garam masala
- 4 teaspoons of ground coriander
- 4 teaspoons of ground peppercorns
- 2 teaspoons of ground ginger
- 2 teaspoons of paprika
- 1 teaspoon of cayenne pepper

For the Chicken:

- 4 whole chickens, cut into 8 pieces each (48 pieces total)
- Canola oil, to coat the griddle
- 8 cups of all-purpose flour
- 8 teaspoons of ground coriander
- 8 teaspoons of garam masala
- 8 teaspoons of ground peppercorns
- 4 teaspoons of ground turmeric
- 2 teaspoons of kosher salt
- 1 teaspoon of cayenne pepper

DIRECTIONS:

1. You'll make the brine first. Mix all the brine ingredients in a big container or pitcher until the salt and sugar are fully dissolved.
2. Get four strong, resealable plastic bags. Split the chicken pieces equally among the bags, then pour half of the brine into each bag.
3. Seal the bags and shake them to make sure the chicken is coated. Place the bags in the fridge and leave them there overnight.
4. Preheat your griddle over medium-high heat and pour in the canola oil.
5. Mix the flour, ground coriander, garam masala, ground peppercorns, ground turmeric, kosher salt, and cayenne pepper in a big bowl.
6. Take a few pieces of chicken out of the brine at a time. Then, coat them in the seasoned flour mixture. Make sure to cover all sides of the chicken and shake off any extra flour.
7. Carefully place the breaded chicken pieces on the flat top in batches. Cook the chicken for 6 to 8 minutes on each side until it's golden brown and fully cooked.
8. Use tongs to move the chicken pieces to a baking sheet lined with paper towels to drain off any excess oil. Repeat the grilling process in batches until all the chicken is cooked.
9. Serve your chicken while it's hot, paired with dipping sauces.

Chapter 11:
Desserts on the Griddle

Many people would agree that dessert is the fun part of every meal, where you indulge in cakes, cookies, ice cream, pies, and other sugary regrettable decisions. But it's dessert, so it's fine, everybody agrees. It is a reward, a celebration of sorts, a chance to satisfy your sweet tooth and put a smile on your face.

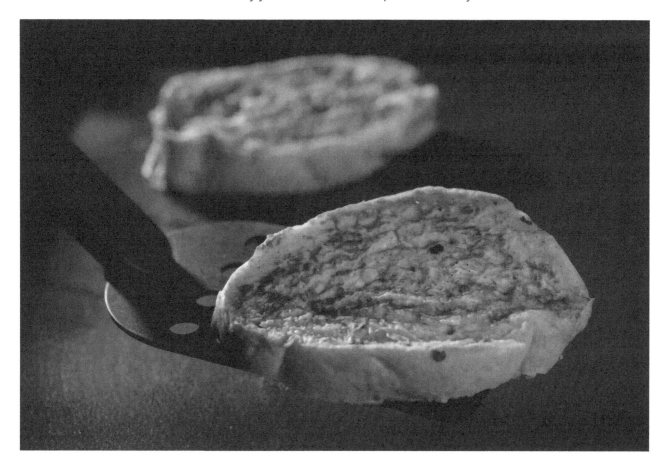

The idea of having a special sweet course at the end of a meal has been around for a really long time. It didn't get "invented" by any one person. It kind of evolved naturally as people's tastes and dining traditions changed over time. These days, the dessert course is as integral to a proper meal as the main dish itself. In fact, you could argue that it's the true star of the show, the grand finale that people are counting down the minutes for. It's the final flourish that takes a meal from great to unforgettable.

The options for dessert on your griddle are just too many to count. It doesn't matter if you're in the mood for something classic and comforting or bold and inventive. Your griddle is sure to rise to the occasion. If you're wondering what kind of desserts you could possibly make on a flat-top griddle, the following recipes could inspire you.

TIPS FOR MAKING DESSERT ON A GAS GRIDDLE
- For ingredients like fruit or cake, slice or dice them into even pieces so they cook at the same rate.
- Don't overcrowd the griddle. Cook desserts in small, manageable batches to maintain temperature control.
- Put down some foil or parchment paper to make cleanup easier, especially for sticky desserts.

- Add toppings, sauces, or garnishes after removing the dessert from the hot griddle.
- Don't be afraid of a little blackening or caramelization.

KITCHEN TOOLS NEEDED

- Mixing bowl
- Parchment paper
- Baking sheet or melting dome
- Aluminum foil
- Basting brush
- Rolling pin
- Bench scraper
- Blender
- Wooden skewers
- Small saucepan
- Cooking spray
- Cookie cutter
- Deep baking dish (10 or 12 inches)
- Serving plates

CINNAMON BISCUITS

Serving: 10
Prep time: 10 mins
Cooking time: 15 mins

INGREDIENTS:

- 2 cans of frozen Grands buttermilk biscuits
- 1 cup of granulated sugar
- 2 tablespoons of ground cinnamon
- 4 tablespoons of melted, unsalted butter

DIRECTIONS:

1. Preheat your griddle on medium-low heat.
2. Get a big bowl and mix the sugar and cinnamon.
3. Get the biscuits and cut each one into quarters, making 48 small pieces.
4. Toss those biscuit pieces in the sugar-cinnamon mix until they're fully coated.
5. You don't want the biscuits to stick and burn, so lay down a big sheet of parchment paper on the preheated griddle.
6. Put the coated biscuit pieces in a single layer on the parchment-lined griddle and drizzle some melted butter over them.
7. Cover the griddle with a lid or a large inverted baking sheet to create a dome and cook for 12 to 15 minutes, flipping them halfway through. The biscuits should be golden brown at the end.
8. Transfer the cooked biscuits to a serving dish and enjoy them warm with a side of cream cheese icing for dipping.

BERRY FOIL PACKETS

Serving: 8
Prep time: 10 mins
Cooking time: 20 mins

INGREDIENTS:

- 5 cups of mixed berries (blueberries, raspberries, blackberries)
- Juice of 1 lemon
- ½ cup of unsalted butter, thawed and cubed
- 3 cups of old-fashioned rolled oats
- 2 tablespoons of all-purpose flour

- ½ cup of brown sugar, divided
- ⅔ cup of chopped pecans
- 2 teaspoons of ground cinnamon
- 1 teaspoon of kosher salt
- Vanilla ice cream for serving (Optional)

DIRECTIONS:

1. Preheat your griddle over medium-high heat.
2. Pour the mixed berries into a bowl with the lemon juice and 2 tablespoons of brown sugar. Toss to mix, and set it aside.
3. Add the oats, flour, pecans, butter, remaining ¼ cup of brown sugar, cinnamon, and salt to a separate bowl. Mix until you get a crumbly mixture.
4. Cut eight 12-inch squares of heavy-duty aluminum foil. Grease the foil squares with a bit of cooking spray.
5. Share the berry mixture among the eight foil squares, placing the berries in the center of each square.
6. Sprinkle the crumble topping over the berry mixture, dividing it among the eight packets.
7. Fold the foil over the filling to create a sealed packet, crimping the edges tightly to prevent any leaks.
8. Place the foil packets on the griddle. Cover the griddle with a lid or melting dome.
9. Cook the berry packets for 15 to 20 minutes.
10. Carefully remove the packets from the griddle and let them cool for a few minutes.
11. Serve the warm berry packets on their own or topped with a scoop of vanilla ice cream.

GRILLED PEACHES

Serving: 24
Prep time: 10 mins
Cooking time: 10 mins

INGREDIENTS:

- 12 ripe peaches, halved and pitted
- 2 tablespoons of vegetable or canola oil
- Vanilla ice cream for serving (optional)
- Honey, for drizzling
- Sea salt

DIRECTIONS:

1. Preheat your griddle to medium-high.
2. Brush the cut side of the peach halves with vegetable or canola oil.
3. Arrange the peach halves, cut side down, on the griddle.
4. Grill the peach halves for 4 or 5 minutes until they are soft and have scorch marks on the cut side.
5. Gently flip the peach halves over so the skin side faces down on the griddle.
6. Grill the peach halves for an extra 4 minutes or until they almost fall apart and are caramelized.
7. Take them off the griddle and onto a serving platter or individual plates.
8. Drizzle the cut sides with honey and sprinkle with a pinch of sea salt.
9. Serve with a scoop of vanilla ice cream.

RICE KRISPIE S'MORES

Serving: 8
Prep time: 10 mins
Cooking time: 7 mins

INGREDIENTS:

- 3 tablespoons of unsalted butter
- ½ teaspoon of kosher salt
- 1 10-ounce pack of marshmallows (any size)
- 6 cups of Rice Krispies cereal
- 6 plain graham crackers
- ⅔ cup of semi-sweet chocolate chips
- ½ cup of mini marshmallows
- Extra mini marshmallows, chocolate chips, graham cracker pieces for garnish (optional)

DIRECTIONS:

1. Crush the graham crackers into large crumbs or chunks and set them aside.
2. Preheat your gas griddle on low heat.
3. Place the butter and salt on the griddle and let it melt, stirring frequently with a spatula so it doesn't burn.
4. Add the marshmallows to the melted butter and continue stirring until the marshmallows have fully melted and are smooth.
5. Immediately add the Rice Krispies to the melted marshmallow mixture, a few cups at a time, mixing it in well with a bench scraper.
6. Once all the cereal is mixed in, stir in the graham cracker crumbs, chocolate pieces, and mini marshmallows.
7. Turn off the heat. Press the Rice Krispie mixture into an even layer on the griddle with your spatula and bench scraper.
8. Let it cool completely before cutting it into squares.
9. Top the squares with extra marshmallows, chocolate, and graham cracker pieces if you want.

SWEET BANANA BITES

Serving: 6
Prep time: 10 mins
Cooking time: 10 mins

INGREDIENTS:

- 6 dinner rolls
- 6 tablespoons of peanut butter
- 6 tablespoons of semi-sweet chocolate chips
- 2 or 3 tablespoons of brown sugar

- 2 medium-sized bananas
- 1 tablespoon of melted butter
- A pinch of salt
- ½ cup of marshmallow creme (optional)

DIRECTIONS:

1. Preheat your griddle to medium-low.
2. Cut the sweet rolls in half horizontally, but don't cut all the way through.
3. Spread 1 tablespoon of peanut butter on the cut side of each roll, then sprinkle 1 tablespoon of chocolate chips on top.
4. Close each roll and wrap each one in a foil packet. Put the packets on the griddle and grill for 3 minutes, flipping halfway to warm both sides of the rolls.
5. While the rolls are warming, peel the bananas and cut each one crosswise into 3 pieces.
6. Pour the brown sugar into a shallow bowl. Coat the banana pieces with the melted butter, then roll them in the brown sugar.
7. Once the rolls are warmed, take the foil packets off the griddle and let them cool.
8. Place the brown sugar-coated banana pieces directly on the hot griddle. Grill them for 3 minutes, turning them a few times to heat all the sides.
9. Take the banana pieces off the griddle and put one inside each warm roll.
10. If you like, top the banana pieces with a small spoonful of marshmallow creme. Close the roll and serve.

BANANA BOATS

Serving: 6
Prep time: 10 mins
Cooking time: 5 mins

INGREDIENTS:

- 6 bananas, with skins
- ¾ cup of semi-sweet chocolate chips
- ¾ cup of marshmallows

DIRECTIONS:

1. Preheat your griddle to medium-low.
2. Take each banana and carefully slice it down the middle without cutting all the way through. You want to make a little boat shape with the banana.
3. Divide the chocolate chips and marshmallows among the 6 banana boats, stuffing the slit in each banana with about 2 tablespoons of chocolate chips and 2 tablespoons of marshmallows.
4. Place the stuffed banana boats on the griddle. Cover the griddle with a lid or melting dome to help the chocolate and marshmallows melt.
5. Cook these banana boats for 5 minutes until the chocolate has melted and the marshmallows are warm and liquid.
6. Use tongs or a spatula to carefully take the banana boats off the griddle once they're done.
7. Let the banana boats cool for a minute, then serve them warm with a spoon to scoop out the chocolate and marshmallow filling.

MANGO AND PINEAPPLE SKEWERS

Serving: 12
Prep time: 10 mins
Cooking time: 10 mins

INGREDIENTS:

- ½ cup of unsalted cashews
- ¾ cup of coconut milk
- 2 tablespoons of honey
- 1 tablespoon of coconut oil

- 1½ cups of coconut flakes
- 1 fresh pineapple, skin removed, diced
- 1 fresh mango, skin removed, diced
- 12 skewers

DIRECTIONS:

1. Soak the cashews in water for 1 or 2 hours, then drain them.
2. Put the soaked cashews, coconut milk, honey, and coconut oil in a blender. Blend until the dip is smooth. Pour the dip into a bowl, cover it, and put it in the fridge.
3. Preheat your griddle to medium-high.
4. Spread the coconut flakes in a single layer on the griddle. Toast the coconut for 2 to 3 minutes until it is golden brown. Take the toasted coconut off the griddle and set it aside.
5. Thread the pineapple and mango cubes onto the skewers.
6. Place the fruit skewers on the griddle. Cook each side for 1 or 2 minutes or until the fruit has a few scorch marks.
7. Remove the grilled fruit skewers from the griddle.
8. Sprinkle the toasted coconut flakes over the chilled coconut milk dip.
9. Serve the warm mango and pineapple skewers with a coconut dip.

PINEAPPLE AND RUM SAUCE SUNDAE

Serving: 4
Prep time: 10 mins
Cooking time: 10 mins

INGREDIENTS:

- 8 slices of fresh pineapple, core removed
- 2 tablespoons of butter
- ¼ cup of brown sugar
- ¼ cup of dark rum
- 2 teaspoons of vanilla extract
- 4 cups of vanilla ice cream
- ¼ cup of shredded sweetened coconut, toasted

DIRECTIONS:

1. Preheat your gas griddle to medium.
2. Place the pineapple slices on the griddle and cook for 3 or 4 minutes per side until they are caramelized with a few scorch marks.
3. Mix the butter, brown sugar, rum, and vanilla in a small saucepan. Cook this on another part of the griddle on low heat. Stir until the sugar has fully melted and the sauce is a dark brown color. Keep the sauce warm.
4. Once the pineapple slices are grilled, place 2 slices each on 4 small plates or bowls.
5. Top each serving with a scoop of vanilla ice cream.
6. Drizzle the warm rum sauce over the ice cream and pineapple.
7. Sprinkle the toasted coconut over the top of the sundaes.

DOUGHNUT AND PEAR SUNDAE

Serving: 4
Prep time: 10 mins
Cooking time: 5 mins

INGREDIENTS:

- 1 tablespoon of sugar
- ¼ teaspoon of cinnamon
- 2 pears, cored and sliced

- 4 glazed doughnuts, split in half
- 4 scoops of vanilla ice cream
- Caramel sauce

DIRECTIONS:

1. Preheat your flat top to medium.
2. Mix the sugar and cinnamon in a bowl. Add the pear slices and toss to coat them in the cinnamon sugar.
3. Place the coated pear slices on the griddle. Grill the pears, turning once, until they are soft and have light scorch marks.
4. Meanwhile, place the split doughnut halves, cut side down, on another spot on the griddle. Grill the doughnuts for just 1 or 2 minutes.
5. For each serving, place one grilled doughnut half on a plate, grilled side up. Top with some of the grilled pear slices, then a scoop of vanilla ice cream.
6. Drizzle the ice cream and pears with a good amount of caramel sauce.
7. Repeat this layering with the remaining doughnut halves, pears, ice cream, and caramel to create 4 grilled doughnut and pear sundaes.
8. Serve this immediately while the doughnuts are still soft and the ice cream is scoopable.

PEACH AND BERRY PIZZA

Serving: 1 pizza
Prep time: 10 mins
Cooking time: 10 mins

INGREDIENTS:

- 2 ounces of softened cream cheese
- 1 (8-ounce) container of crème fraîche
- 3 tablespoons of honey
- ¼ teaspoon of orange zest
- 1 tablespoon of orange juice
- ¼ teaspoon of ground cinnamon

- 1 lb. pizza dough
- 1 peach, halved and pitted
- 1 cup of blackberries
- 1 cup of raspberries
- Torn mint leaves for garnish
- Honey for drizzling

DIRECTIONS:

1. Preheat your griddle to medium-high.
2. Get a small bowl and beat the cream cheese until it's smooth. Then mix in the crème fraîche, honey, orange zest, orange juice, and cinnamon. Stir it properly. Put this mixture in the fridge until you're ready to use it.
3. Roll or stretch out the pizza dough into a 12-inch circle. Brush a light coating of oil over the griddle's surface, then place the dough round on it.
4. Cook the pizza dough for 3 minutes per side, with a lid, until it's toasted and cooked through. Take the grilled crust off the griddle and keep it for later.
5. Put the peach halves, cut side down, on the griddle. Close the lid and cook them for 2 minutes so that they soften and develop scorch marks. Let the peach halves cool, then slice them.
6. Spread the chilled crème fraîche mixture over the now-warm pizza crust.
7. Top this with the sliced grilled peaches, blackberries, and raspberries.
8. Sprinkle some mint leaves and drizzle a little extra honey over it.
9. Slice your dessert pizza and serve right away.

CHEESECAKE QUESADILLA

Serving: 8
Prep time: 10 mins
Cooking time: 10 mins

INGREDIENTS:

- Strawberry syrup
- 8 ounces of softened cream cheese
- ½ cup of powdered sugar
- 1 teaspoon of vanilla extract

- 8 flour tortillas
- Butter
- Cinnamon-sugar mixture
- Whipped cream (Optional)

DIRECTIONS:

1. Mix the softened cream cheese, powdered sugar, and vanilla extract.
2. Preheat your griddle to medium.
3. Butter one side of 4 of the flour tortillas. Sprinkle the buttered side of each tortilla with the cinnamon-sugar mix.
4. Spread half of the cheesecake filling mixture on one side of the remaining unbuttered 4 tortillas.
5. Place one of the buttered, cinnamon-sugar tortillas on top of a filling-topped tortilla, butter side down.
6. Place the quesadilla on the griddle. Add a small pat of butter to the top tortilla and sprinkle with more cinnamon-sugar.
7. Cook both sides of the quesadilla until the tortillas are golden brown.
8. Take the cheesecake quesadilla off the griddle and slice it into 4 or 8 triangles.
9. Top the warm quesadilla slices with the prepared strawberry syrup and a dollop of whipped cream.
10. Repeat steps 7 to 9 to make more cheesecake quesadillas.

FRUIT EMPANADAS

Serving: 10
Prep time: 20 mins
Cooking time: 10 mins

INGREDIENTS:

- 2 cups of flour
- ½ cup plus 1 tablespoon of cooking oil
- 1 teaspoon of baking powder
- 1 teaspoon of ground cinnamon
- 1 teaspoon of sugar
- 2 cups of any fresh or canned fruit, skin off (blueberries, raspberries, strawberries, bananas and apples are good examples)
- ½ cup of brown sugar or fructose
- 2 teaspoons of ground cinnamon
- ½ teaspoon of ground cloves
- ½ teaspoon of ground nutmeg
- Cinnamon sugar, for dusting

DIRECTIONS:

1. Preheat your griddle over medium heat and spray with a light sheen of cooking spray.
2. Mix the flour, ½ cup of oil, baking powder, 1 teaspoon of cinnamon, and sugar in a bowl until a soft dough forms. Add a tiny bit of water if needed to make the dough smooth and silky.
3. Roll out the dough into a fairly thin circle on a flour-dusted surface. Use a 4-inch cookie cutter or biscuit cutter to cut the dough into circles.
4. In a smaller bowl, cut or mash the fruit and add brown sugar, 2 teaspoons of cinnamon, cloves, and nutmeg. Stir to mix.
5. Place one-half of each dough circle with roughly two tablespoons of the fruit filling on it. To create a half-moon shape, fold the remaining dough over the filling. Crimp and seal the edges with a fork.
6. Brush the top of each empanada with the remaining 1 tablespoon of oil.
7. Place the filled and sealed empanadas on the griddle. Cook for 3 to 4 minutes on each side until the dough is golden brown.
8. Take the grilled empanadas off the griddle and immediately sprinkle them with cinnamon sugar.

NUTELLA AND BANANA SANDWICH

Serving: 2
Prep time: 5 mins
Cooking time: 5 mins

INGREDIENTS:

- 4 slices of bread
- 4 tablespoons of Nutella
- 1 ripe banana
- Butter, for grilling

DIRECTIONS:

1. Peel the banana and cut it into rounds.
2. Take 2 slices of bread and spread a bit of Nutella on each slice.
3. Arrange the banana rounds on top of the Nutella on one of the bread slices.
4. Place the other Nutella-spread bread slice on top to make a sandwich.
5. Preheat your griddle to medium.
6. Butter the outside of the sandwich on one side.
7. Place the sandwich on the griddle butter-side down. Butter the top side while the bottom cooks. In 2 minutes, flip it and cook the other side for another 2 minutes.
8. Repeat steps 2 to 7 to make more sandwiches.

Chapter 12:

Vegetarian and Vegan Options

Being a vegetarian or vegan used to mean settling for sad salads and flavorless tofu, but thankfully, the days of deprivation and sacrifice are well in the past. Innovative chefs and food brands have really stepped up their game, pushing the boundaries of what's possible with plant-based ingredients.

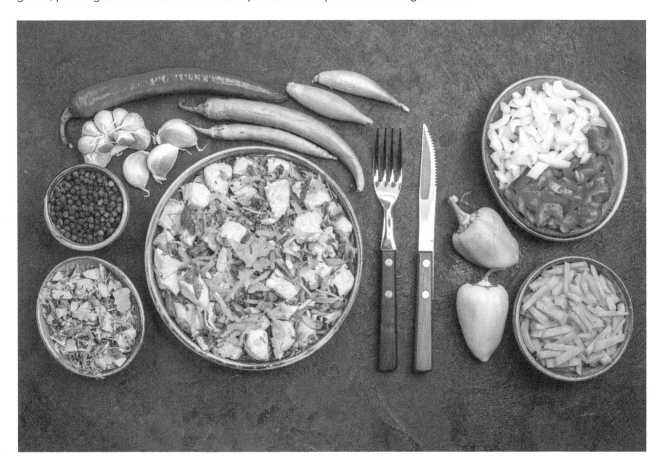

Today, you can find plant-based options that rival anything made with meat or dairy—meatless burgers that bleed, vegan cheese that actually melts, and chicken nuggets made from thin air (or at least some very clever plant materials).

Vegan restaurant. Don't worry about getting across town to that one elusive vegan deli, not when you have a gas griddle. Plant-based recipes are not complicated or time-consuming. With the incredible products and resources available today, it's never been easier. Throw in a little creativity, and there's nothing you can't cook.

TIPS FOR MAKING VEGAN AND VEGETARIAN MEALS ON A GAS GRIDDLE
- Toss mushrooms in a little oil and soy sauce or liquid aminos before grilling to really bring out their umami flavor.
- Get a good sear on plant-based proteins by letting them sit undisturbed on the griddle for 2 to 3 minutes before flipping.
- Use the extra-firm kind of tofu. This is the best type for grilling because it's sturdy and won't fall apart on the griddle.

- Deglaze the griddle with a splash of broth, wine, or vinegar to scrape up any browned bits and use as a sauce.
- Use a spray bottle filled with water to mist the griddle if ingredients start to stick or char too quickly.

KITCHEN TOOLS NEEDED

- Mixing bowl
- Potato masher
- Rolling pin
- Cooking spray
- Baking sheet
- Melting dome
- Peeler
- Ziplock bag
- Vegetable spiralizer
- Large metal pot or pan
- Small metal pot
- Food processor
- Basting brush
- Box grater
- Paper towels
- Wooden skewers
- Tofu press

PESTO PIZZA

Serving: 1 pizza
Prep time: 10 mins
Cooking time: 10 mins

INGREDIENTS:

- ½ cup of white whole-wheat flour
- ¾ teaspoon of instant yeast
- ¼ teaspoon of pure cane sugar
- A dash of sea salt
- 1 (7½ oz) can of unsalted cannellini beans, rinsed and drained
- 1 teaspoon of lemon juice
- ¼ cup of homemade vegan pesto
- ¼ of a yellow bell pepper, cut into thin strips
- 1 tablespoon of chopped red onion
- ¾ cup of cherry tomatoes, halved
- Crushed red pepper (Optional)

DIRECTIONS:

1. Mix the flour, yeast, sugar, and salt in a bowl. Add ¼ cup of warm water and stir until you get a soft dough.
2. On a flour-dusted surface, knead the dough for 2 or 3 minutes until it's smooth and stretchy.
3. Mash the beans, lemon juice, and 1 teaspoon of water in another bowl until it is nearly smooth.
4. Roll the dough into a flat oval shape.
5. Heat your griddle over medium heat and spray with cooking oil.
6. Carefully place the dough oval onto the hot griddle. Cook for 2 or 3 minutes with the lid closed until the bottom is browned.
7. Transfer the crust to a lightly oiled baking sheet, browned side up. Spread the bean mixture over the crust, then spread the vegan pesto on top.
8. Add the bell pepper strips, onion, and tomatoes as toppings.
9. Slide the topped pizza back onto the griddle. Cook for another 3 minutes with a lid or melting dome until the bottom is browned.
10. Remove the pizza from the griddle and cut it into wedges. Sprinkle with crushed red pepper, and serve.

CARROT DOGS

Serving: 2
Prep time: 4 hrs 10 mins
Cooking time: 10 mins

INGREDIENTS:

- 2 large carrots
- 1 tablespoon of apple cider vinegar
- ¼ cup of low-sodium vegetable broth
- 2 whole wheat hot dog buns, toasted
- 1½ teaspoons of reduced-sodium soy sauce or tamari
- 1 teaspoon of smoked paprika
- 1 teaspoon of dry mustard
- 1½ teaspoons of maple syrup

- 1½ tablespoons of stone-ground mustard
- ¼ teaspoon of ground coriander
- ¼ teaspoon of onion powder
- ¼ teaspoon of liquid smoke
- ¼ teaspoon of garlic powder
- Dash of ground cloves
- 2 tablespoons of chopped red onion
- ¼ of a medium cucumber, spiralized

DIRECTIONS:

1. Peel the carrots and trim them to 6 inches long. Trim the wide ends to make the thickness more uniform.
2. Pour the vegetable broth, apple cider vinegar, soy sauce, maple syrup, smoked paprika, dry mustard, ground coriander, garlic powder, onion powder, liquid smoke, and a dash of ground cloves into a bowl. Add ¼ cup of water and stir to mix.
3. Place the carrots in a resealable plastic bag and pour the marinade over them. Seal the bag and refrigerate for 4 to 24 hours, shaking the bag every now and then.
4. Preheat your griddle over medium-high heat. Drain the carrots and discard the marinade.
5. Place the marinated carrots on the griddle and cook for 5 to 8 minutes until you see scorch marks.
6. Remove the grilled carrots and place them in the toasted hot dog buns.
7. Top each carrot dog with 1 tablespoon chopped red onion, ¾ tablespoon stone-ground mustard, and some spiralized cucumber.

TOMATO AND ZUCCHINI SLIDERS

Serving: 4
Prep time: 30 mins
Cooking time: 26 mins

INGREDIENTS:

- ½ cup of chopped onion
- ½ cup of coarsely chopped fresh mushrooms
- 1 minced garlic clove
- ¾ cup of cooked chickpeas (about ¼ cup of dry chickpeas, cooked)
- 2 tablespoons of chickpea cooking liquid (aquafaba)
- ¼ cup of chopped sun-dried tomatoes (not oil-packed)

- 1 teaspoon of Italian seasoning, crushed
- ½ teaspoon of lemon zest
- Sea salt and ground black pepper for seasoning
- 2 tablespoons of cornmeal
- 1 medium zucchini, cut lengthwise into ½-inch thick planks
- 1 tablespoon of balsamic vinegar
- 4 small Roma tomato slices

DIRECTIONS:

1. On the griddle set to low heat, cook the chopped onion, mushrooms, and garlic over medium heat for 3 to 4 minutes. Stir and add a little water if it starts to stick.
2. Transfer the cooked vegetable mixture to a food processor. Add the cooked chickpeas, 2 tablespoons of the chickpea cooking liquid, the chopped sun-dried tomatoes, Italian seasoning, and lemon zest. Pulse it a few times until the mixture is chunky but not completely smooth. If it seems a little dry, add 1 or 2 more tablespoons of the chickpea liquid.
3. With wet hands, shape the chickpea mixture into 4 small patties. Put the patties in the fridge for at least 20 minutes to get firm.
4. Coat the chilled patties all over with the cornmeal.
5. Preheat your griddle to medium-high.
6. Cook the chickpea patties on the griddle for 8 to 10 minutes, flipping them once so they're browned on both sides and heated through.
7. While the patties cook, brush the zucchini slices with the balsamic vinegar. Cook both sides of the zucchini slices on the griddle for 4 to 6 minutes until they're tender-crisp with some burn marks.
8. Cut each zucchini slice into 4 pieces to use as the "buns" for the sliders.
9. Assemble the sliders by putting a chickpea patty and a tomato slice between two pieces of the grilled zucchini. Drizzle with any leftover balsamic vinegar.

PEACH AND BURRATA CROSTINI

Serving: 8
Prep time: 10 mins
Cooking time: 12 mins

INGREDIENTS:

- 1 small French bread loaf
- 1 ripe peach
- Olive oil
- 4 ounces of burrata cheese

- Kosher salt
- Ground black pepper
- Balsamic glaze
- Fresh basil, chopped

DIRECTIONS:

1. Slice the French loaf into 8 pieces.
2. Remove the pit from the peach and cut it into 8 pieces.
3. Preheat your griddle on medium-low heat.
4. Brush both sides of the bread slices and the peach slices with a little olive oil.
5. Place the oiled bread slices and peach slices on the griddle. Cook them for 2 to 3 minutes per side to toast them.
6. Take the toasted bread and peach slices off the griddle. Take the burrata and tear it up, placing it on top of the slices of bread.
7. Put a slice of the grilled peach on top of the burrata on each piece of bread.
8. Sprinkle a little pinch of salt and pepper over the crostini.
9. Put the crostini back on the griddle and cook for 3 more minutes to warm everything through.
10. Remove the crostini from the griddle and drizzle balsamic glaze over the top.
11. Sprinkle with chopped fresh basil, and serve.

BANG BANG RAMEN SAUCE

Serving: 2
Prep time: 10 mins
Cooking time: 20 mins

INGREDIENTS:

- 2 packages of ramen noodles (any flavor, discard the flavor pack or save it for another recipe if you like)
- 3 or 4 tablespoons of Japanese mayo or regular mayo
- 4 tablespoons of sweet Thai chili sauce
- 1 or 2 teaspoons of sriracha (adjust to your spice preference)

- 2 teaspoons of cooking oil
- 4 tablespoons of diced onion
- 1 or 2 minced cloves of garlic
- Kosher salt and black pepper for seasoning
- 3 tablespoons of sliced green onions
- 2 teaspoons of lemon juice

DIRECTIONS:

1. Bring a small pot of water to a boil on the griddle. Cook the ramen noodles according to package directions, but do not add the flavor packets. Drain the noodles and rinse them very well with cold water to prevent them from getting mushy.
2. Mix the mayo, sweet chili sauce, and sriracha in a bowl. This is your bang bang sauce.
3. Your flat top should be preheated over medium heat. Let it get really hot.
4. Add the cooking oil. Follow with the diced onion, and cook for 1 or 2 minutes to soften it.
5. Add the minced garlic, a pinch of kosher salt, and a pinch of black pepper. Stir and cook for 30 seconds.
6. Add the cooked ramen noodles. Use tongs or spatulas to stir and flip the noodles for 2 to 3 minutes until it heats through.
7. Pour half of the bang bang sauce over the noodles and continue cooking and stirring for 3 more minutes.
8. Add the sliced green onions and lemon juice. Stir and cook again for 2 more minutes.
9. Turn off the heat and toss the noodles with the remaining bang bang sauce.

YELLOW SQUASH FRITTERS

Serving: 4
Prep time: 20 mins
Cooking time: 10 mins

INGREDIENTS:

- 1 medium-sized yellow squash
- 1 small shallot, minced
- 1 egg, beaten
- 2 tablespoons of panko breadcrumbs
- ¼ cup of all-purpose flour
- 1½ tablespoons of grated parmesan cheese
- 1 teaspoon of chopped chives

- 1 teaspoon of Old Bay seasoning
- Tabasco sauce
- 1 or 2 tablespoons of cooking oil

Dipping Sauces:
- Spicy mayo
- Sour cream

DIRECTIONS:

1. Get a box grater and shred the yellow squash.
2. Pour the shredded squash onto paper towels in a single layer and leave it for a few minutes.
3. Wrap the squash in the paper towels and squeeze it to get rid of the extra moisture.
4. Mix the shredded squash, minced shallot, beaten egg, panko breadcrumbs, flour, parmesan cheese, chives, and Old Bay seasoning. Add a few dashes of Tabasco sauce if you're feeling up to it. Let the mixture sit for 10 minutes.
5. Scoop out some of the squash mixture and shape it into 4 fritters. Place them on a plate or tray.
6. Preheat your griddle to medium and add 1 or 2 tablespoons of cooking oil.
7. Place the squash fritters on the griddle and press down gently to flatten them. Cook both sides of each fritter for 2 or 3 minutes until golden brown.
8. After that, take them off the griddle and serve them warm. If you want, you can have some sour cream or spicy mayo on the side for dipping.

HIBACHI GARLIC RAMEN NOODLES

Serving: 2
Prep time: 10 mins
Cooking time: 15 mins

INGREDIENTS:

- 2 packs of ramen noodles (throw away the flavor packets or save them for a future recipe)
- 1 or 2 teaspoons of any cooking oil
- ½ medium onion, diced
- 3 to 5 cloves garlic, minced
- 1 tablespoon of hoisin sauce

- 1 tablespoon of soy sauce
- 2 tablespoons of unsalted butter
- 1 egg
- ¼ cup of chopped cilantro or green onions
- Sesame seeds, yum yum sauce, sriracha (Optional)

DIRECTIONS:

1. Bring a saucepan of water to a boil. Cook the ramen noodles according to the package, but don't use the flavor packet. Drain the noodles and rinse them with cold water.
2. Preheat your flat top over medium heat. It should be very hot.
3. Add a small drizzle of cooking oil to the griddle. Then add the diced onion. Cook the onion for 2 or 3 minutes, stirring it with a spatula.
4. Add the minced garlic and cook for about 45 seconds, until it smells fragrant.
5. Add the cooked ramen noodles, hoisin sauce, soy sauce, and butter to the garlic and onions. Use your spatulas to mix and toss everything together.
6. Make a little space in the middle of the noodles, and crack the egg right into that spot. Let the egg cook for 1 or 2 minutes.
7. Keep cooking and stirring the noodles for 5 minutes max, until it's heated through and the egg is cooked.
8. Turn off the heat and stir in the chopped cilantro or green onions. Taste it and add a little more hoisin or soy sauce if you want.
9. Serve with sesame seeds, yum yum sauce, or sriracha.

TEMPEH PINEAPPLE KEBABS WITH PEANUT SATAY SAUCE

Serving: 2
Prep time: 30 mins
Cooking time: 25 mins

INGREDIENTS:

Peanut Satay Sauce:

- ¼ cup of peanut butter
- ¼ cup of olive oil
- ½ cup of coconut milk
- 1 tablespoon of tamari soy sauce
- 1 minced clove of garlic
- 1 tablespoon of apple cider vinegar
- ½ teaspoon of grated ginger
- Sea salt, for seasoning

- A dash of red pepper flakes

Kebabs:

- Whole pineapple
- 4 ounces of tempeh, original or multigrain, cut into 12 (1-inch) cubes
- ½ small red onion
- 1 tablespoon of tamari soy sauce
- 6 (12-inch) skewers, metal, or soaked wooden

DIRECTIONS:

1. Pour the olive oil, peanut butter, coconut milk, soy sauce, vinegar, garlic, ginger, and red pepper flakes into a blender. Blend it until the sauce is smooth. Taste it and add a pinch of salt if you need to. Pour the sauce into a bowl.
2. Put the tempeh cubes in a small pot on the griddle and add just enough water to cover them. Stir in the soy sauce. Let the water boil, then turn the heat down and let it simmer for 5 minutes, stirring the tempeh once.
3. Drain the tempeh and add it to the bowl with the peanut sauce. Toss the tempeh in the sauce to coat it. Let it sit while you prepare the pineapple and onion.
4. Slice off the skin of the pineapple, cutting deep enough to remove most of the little pineapple eyes.
5. Cut the pineapple into 12 cubes that are about 1 inch big. Peel the onion and cut it into 12 wedges that are also 1 inch thick.
6. Preheat your griddle to medium-high.
7. Start threading the skewers, alternating between the onion wedges, pineapple cubes, and tempeh cubes. Put an onion wedge at the beginning and end of each skewer.
8. Put the skewered kebabs on the griddle. Use a spoon or brush to coat the kebabs with the peanut sauce. Cook for 18 to 20 minutes, turning the kebabs and brushing them with more sauce every so often. You want to get some scorch marks on the tempeh and pineapple.
9. Serve the kebabs right away. Put any extra peanut sauce on the side for dipping. You can serve the kebabs with some steamed brown rice or quinoa.

BREADED TOFU

Serving: 4
Prep time: 1 hr 10 mins
Cooking time: 20 mins

INGREDIENTS:

Tofu Marinade:

- 10 ounces of extra firm tofu
- 2 teaspoons of low-sodium tamari or soy sauce
- ½ teaspoon of maple syrup
- 1½ tablespoons of ketchup
- ¼ teaspoon of hot sauce (Optional)
- ¼ teaspoon of garam masala (or ¼ teaspoon of ground cumin and ¼ teaspoon of ground coriander)
- 1 teaspoon of oil

- A dash of salt
- ¼ teaspoon of garlic powder
- ¼ teaspoon of cornstarch or tapioca starch (Optional)

Breadcrumb Coating:

- ½ cup of breadcrumbs (use gluten-free if you like)
- ¼ teaspoon of cayenne pepper
- A dash of salt
- 1 teaspoon of nutritional yeast (Optional)

DIRECTIONS:

1. Take the block of tofu. Use some paper towels or a tofu press to press out any extra water from the tofu for about 30 minutes.
2. Cut the pressed tofu into 12 long, rectangular strips.
3. Mix the soy sauce, ketchup, maple syrup, hot sauce, oil, garam masala (or cumin and coriander), garlic powder, salt, and cornstarch or tapioca starch in a shallow bowl. Add the tofu strips and gently toss them around to coat all the sides with the marinade. Cover the bowl and put it in the fridge for at least 30 minutes.
4. Mix the breadcrumbs, a pinch of salt, a pinch or two of cayenne pepper, and the nutritional yeast in another shallow bowl.
5. Preheat your flat top to medium-high.
6. Take each marinated tofu strip and dip it into the breadcrumb mixture, coating all the sides.
7. Lightly oil the griddle and place the breaded tofu strips on it.
8. Cook the breaded tofu for 7 to 9 minutes per side or until you see golden brown marks on both sides.
9. Serve with your favorite dipping sauces, or use them in salads, wraps, and sandwiches.

SHIITAKE AND TOFU BANH MI

Serving: 2
Prep time: 30 mins
Cooking time: 10 mins

INGREDIENTS:

- 7 ounces of extra-firm tofu
- 2 tablespoons plus 1 teaspoon of distilled white vinegar
- 1 teaspoon of sugar
- Kosher salt
- 1 medium carrot, skin shaved
- ½ English cucumber, thinly sliced on the bias and then sliced in half
- 2 tablespoons of mayonnaise
- ¼ to ½ teaspoon of Sriracha

- 1 grated clove of garlic
- ½ cup of hoisin sauce
- 1 tablespoon of vegetable oil, plus more for oiling the griddle
- 8 ounces of large-capped shiitake mushrooms, stems removed
- Ground black pepper
- 2 soft hoagie rolls, sliced almost all the way through lengthwise
- ½ cup of fresh cilantro

DIRECTIONS:

1. Take the block of extra-firm tofu and place it between two plates. If you don't have a tofu press, put any heavy object on top of the top plate, like a can or a skillet, to press down on the tofu for about 20 minutes. This will squeeze out any extra water in the tofu.
2. Mix 2 tablespoons of the white vinegar, ¼ cup of water, the sugar, and a pinch of salt until the sugar and salt have dissolved. Add the shredded carrot and sliced cucumber, toss everything, and put the bowl in the fridge until you're ready to assemble the sandwiches.
3. Get another bowl, and mix the mayonnaise and a little bit of the Sriracha sauce. Set this aside.
4. After the tofu has been pressed, pat it dry and cut it into 4 slices that are a half-inch thick.
5. Get yet another bowl and mix the grated garlic, the hoisin sauce, the remaining 1 teaspoon of vinegar, and 1 tablespoon of oil. Add the mushroom caps and toss to coat the mushrooms.
6. Preheat your griddle on medium-high heat and spray the surface lightly with cooking oil.
7. Remove the mushroom caps from the marinade, shake off any extra, and place them on the hot griddle. Cook for about 1 minute, flipping them once until they're charred. Then flip them and cook for 30 seconds to 1 minute more until they're almost soft. Move the cooked mushrooms to a plate.
8. Toss the tofu slices in the remaining mushroom marinade.

9. Put the tofu slices on the griddle, with the marinated side down, and cook for 2 minutes. Flip them and cook the other side for 2 more minutes.

10. While the tofu is cooking, toast the open-faced rolls on another spot on the griddle for 2 minutes.

11. Spread 1 heaping tablespoon of the mayonnaise-sriracha mixture on each half of the toasted rolls. Place 2 pieces of the cooked tofu on each roll, then top with the grilled mushroom slices, overlapping them a bit.

12. Add some of the chilled carrot and cucumber salad on top, and sprinkle on some fresh cilantro.

13. Close up the sandwiches, pressing them down gently, and serve.

EGGPLANT AND CHICKPEA WRAPS

Serving: 2
Prep time: 20 mins
Cooking time: 5 mins

INGREDIENTS:

- 1 small clove of garlic
- 1 teaspoon of fresh lemon juice
- 6 tablespoons of Greek yogurt
- Kosher salt
- 1 (15.5 oz) can of chickpeas, rinsed, drained, and patted dry
- 1 small eggplant, sliced into 7 thick rounds
- 2 tablespoons of olive oil

- 2 (10-inch) soft tortillas
- 2 teaspoons of dried oregano
- 1 small tomato, diced (roughly 4 oz)
- 1 small Persian cucumber, quartered lengthwise and thinly sliced (roughly 2 oz)
- ¼ small head of romaine, thinly sliced (about ½ cup)

DIRECTIONS:

1. Preheat your griddle on medium-high heat.
2. Grate the garlic clove into a bowl. Squeeze in the lemon juice and let that sit for 2 minutes. Then whisk in the Greek yogurt, 1 tablespoon of water, and a pinch of salt.
3. Add the drained and dried chickpeas to another bowl and stir in 2 tablespoons of the garlic-yogurt sauce. Keep this for later.
4. Slice the eggplant into 7 thick rounds. Brush one side of the eggplant slices with 1 tablespoon of olive oil and sprinkle them with a little salt.
5. Place the oiled side of the eggplant slices down on the griddle and grill them for 2 minutes.
6. Brush the tops of the eggplant slices with the remaining 1 tablespoon of olive oil, sprinkle them with a bit more salt, flip them over, and grill for 2 more minutes until they're very soft.
7. Take the grilled eggplant slices off the griddle and roughly chop them. Stir the chopped eggplant into the bowl with the chickpea mixture. Taste it and add a pinch more salt if you want.
8. Grab the tortillas. Spread 2 tablespoons of the garlic-yogurt sauce onto each one, then sprinkle 1 teaspoon of oregano over the sauce.
9. Scoop half of the chickpea-eggplant mixture and form it into a log across the center of each tortilla, leaving 1 inch of space on the sides.

10. Top the chickpea-eggplant mixture with half the diced tomato, a pinch of salt, some sliced cucumber, and a small handful of the shredded romaine.

11. Fold the sides of the tortilla over the ends of the filling, then tightly roll up the tortilla from the bottom to make a wrap.

12. Repeat steps 9 to 11 with the remaining tortilla and filling.

13. Cut each wrap in half diagonally and serve.

BBQ TEMPEH

Serving: 4
Prep time: 10 mins
Cooking time: 25 mins

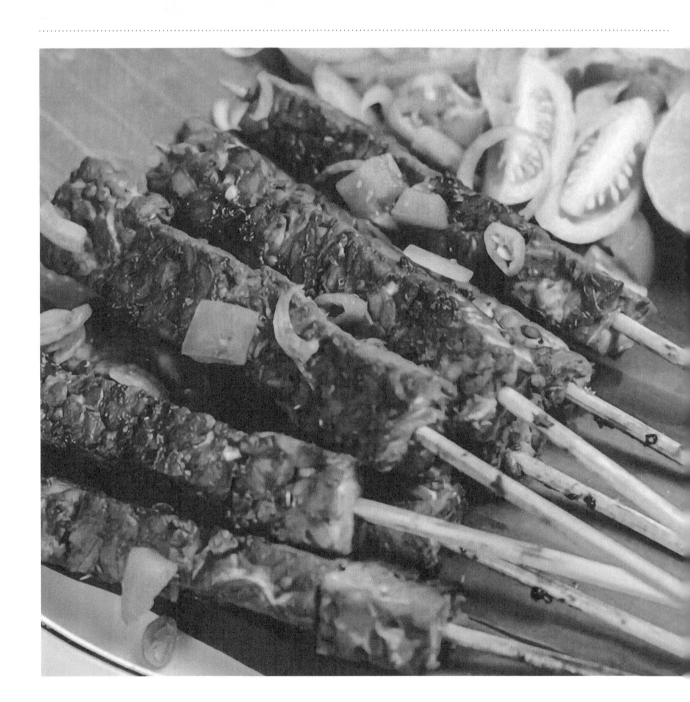

INGREDIENTS:

- ⅓ cup of water, plus more as necessary
- 5 tablespoons of soy sauce
- 1½ tablespoons of maple syrup
- 1½ teaspoons of liquid smoke
- 1½ teaspoons of sweet paprika
- ¾ teaspoon of onion powder
- ¾ teaspoon of garlic powder
- 1 (12 oz) package of tempeh
- 1½ tablespoons of canola oil
- 1½ cups of vegan barbecue sauce, divided

DIRECTIONS:

1. Mix the water, soy sauce, maple syrup, liquid smoke, paprika, onion powder, and garlic powder in a bowl.
2. Take the whole block of tempeh and place it in a medium to large-sized pan. Pour the soy sauce mixture over the top of the tempeh.
3. Put the pan on the griddle over medium heat and let the liquid gently simmer. The tempeh should simmer for 5 minutes before you flip it and let it simmer for 5 more minutes. Use a spoon to scoop some of the liquid over the tempeh every now and then. If the liquid starts to dry up, add a splash of more water to the pan.
4. After the tempeh has simmered for 10 minutes, take it out of the pan.
5. Put your griddle on medium-high. Add the canola oil.
6. Once the oil is hot, add the block of tempeh. Let it cook for 5 minutes per side until it's browned and crispy on the outside.
7. Take the cooked tempeh off the griddle and put it on a plate. Use a brush or spoon to spread ¾ cup of the barbecue sauce all over the top and sides of the tempeh.
8. Place the sauced tempeh back on the griddle. Grill for 8 minutes or until you see some charred spots.
9. Take it off the heat and slice it into 12 long strips.
10. Serve the BBQ tempeh warm, with the remaining barbecue sauce on the side.

Chapter 13:
Advanced Techniques and Recipes

By now, you've mastered the basics of griddle cooking, so it's time to level up and really start impressing your friends, family, and taste buds. The first, and arguably the most important, skill here is getting the perfect sear. The perfect sear is the holy grail. It is that golden-brown crust on the outside that doesn't just look nice but overflows with so much savory, caramelized flavor. It is the whole point of grilling in the first place.

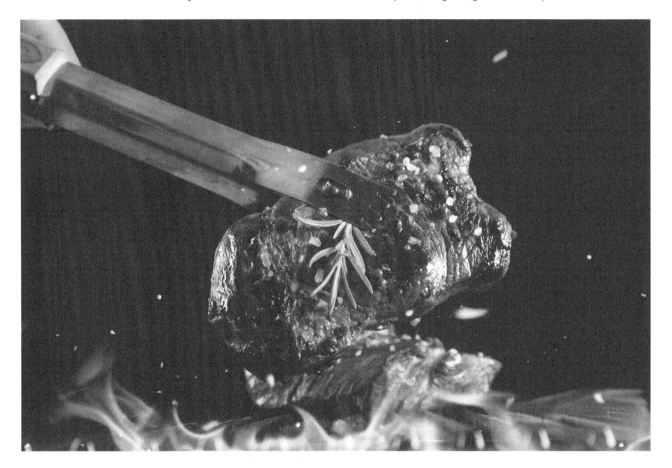

GETTING THE PERFECT SEAR

You need to start with a ripping hot griddle to get that perfect sear. This intense temperature is important for quickly browning the surface before the inside overcooks. This intense heat is also what kickstarts the Maillard reaction, the chemical process that transforms the sugars and amino acids in the food into hundreds of amazing flavor compounds. That's where that trademark brown color and crackly texture come from. But it's not just the heat here. You also want that surface to be dry. That means the food has to be bone dry before it even hits the griddle. Any leftover moisture will create steam, and that's the enemy of a good sear. So pat your proteins and vegetables down with paper towels until they're as dry as a bone.

The tricky part of getting the perfect sear is timing it just right. You only need a couple of minutes on each side to get those beautiful scorch marks. Any longer and you risk burning the outside while the center is still undercooked. The real test of your searing skills, though, is restraint. It takes the willpower and patience of a saint not to poke and prod at your food as it cooks. Those critical minutes of undisturbed searing time allow that crust to develop into something truly special. Just let it be, and you'll know it's time to behold your handiwork when the food releases from the griddle effortlessly.

SMOKING AND FLAVORING

Smoking is the process of infusing food with a smoky, almost barbecue-like flavor and smell. This is done by exposing the food to smoke from smoldering wood chips or other sources of smoke. The smoke contains compounds that adhere to the surface of the food, giving it that distinct smoky taste. With your gas griddle, there are a few easy ways to do this:

- **Wood chips:** Burn some dry wood chips (like hickory, mesquite, or apple) in an aluminum foil pan beside your food on the griddle. Cover them both with a lid and put the heat on low. As they smoke, the flavor will transfer to your food.
- **Liquid smoke:** Brush or drizzle a little liquid smoke seasoning onto your food as it cooks.

Whichever smoky route you choose, start light and gradually work your way up until you find your ideal balance of burnt-to-a-crisp and "mmm, that's the stuff." Conversely, flavoring involves techniques used to imbue food with extra tastes and aromas beyond the base ingredients. This involves applying dry seasonings, marinating in liquids, basting with sauces, or using compound butters.

- **Dry rubs:** A dry rub is just a mix of dried spices, herbs, salts, and other seasonings you rub or pat onto your food. You can use any dried spice, for example, paprika, garlic powder, onion powder, chili powder, brown sugar, black pepper, etc. For this to work, you need to coat all sides of the food. The high heat of the griddle will then make the seasonings caramelize, giving the outside of the food a tasty crust.
- **Marinades:** Marinades are liquid seasoning mixtures in which you soak your food before cooking. This tenderizes the food and infuses it with an extra dimension of taste. A marinade could contain ingredients like vinegar, citrus juice, or wine, as well as herbs, spices, garlic, and oil. You let the food sit in the marinade in the fridge for anywhere from 30 minutes to 24 hours. This gives the flavors time to really soak in. Cooking marinated food caramelizes the seasonings and blends them with the natural flavors of whatever you marinate to give you layers and layers of flavor.
- **Basting sauces:** Basting is the process of brushing or spooning a sauce or liquid over food as it cooks, usually towards the end of the cooking process. Your options for this include barbecue sauce, melted butter or oil, wine, fruit juices, and even marinades. Try not to over-baste your food, though, because it will just get soggy. Instead, brush or spoon the sauce on top of the food every few minutes or in the last minutes of cooking, depending on the recipe.

TIPS FOR USING MARINADES AND RUBS

- Use sugary marinades carefully because they could burn and leave a bitter taste in your food.
- Give your rubs at least 30 minutes to sit before you start cooking. This lets the flavors develop.
- For thin meats or seafood, marinate for 30 minutes to an hour. Thicker foods may need 2 to 4 hours or more.
- Use a bowl that's big enough. You want room to toss the ingredients around, not just a bowl that barely contains the protein.
- Clean your griddle very well between batches so flavors don't carry over unless you want them to.
- Apply rubs in multiple thin layers rather than one thick coating so they stick better.

- Make sure your meat is dry before marinating. Blot it with paper towels until it is completely dry. Extra moisture will water down the flavor and make it harder to get a good sear on the griddle.
- Try doing a dry brine on the meat before you pat on the rub. The salt will season the interior and retain moisture.
- Use a marinade with ingredients like pineapple, papaya, or kiwi for tougher meats. They have enzymes that will break down and tenderize the meat.
- For seafood, use a citrus-based marinade to keep the flesh firm while it cooks.
- Do both a marinade and a dry rub for a double-layered flavor profile.

BARBECUE RUB

INGREDIENTS:

- ⅓ cup of dark brown sugar
- 1 tablespoon of granulated onion powder
- 4 teaspoons of ground mustard
- ⅓ cup of paprika
- 2 teaspoons of ground black pepper

- 1 tablespoon of granulated garlic powder
- 2 teaspoons of ground coriander seeds
- 1 tablespoon of dried oregano
- ¼ cup of kosher salt

DIRECTIONS:

1. Preheat your griddle over medium heat and make sure it's very dry.
2. Toast the ground mustard, black pepper, and coriander for 2 to 3 minutes or until fragrant. This step is to bring out the flavors of these spices.
3. Pour all the prepared spices and seasonings into a bowl. Use your fingertips to break up any large clumps of brown sugar.
4. Mix the ingredients with a whisk until you get a thoroughly blended spice.
5. Pour the barbecue rub into an airtight container and store it at room temperature for up to 4 months. The rub may gradually lose its flavor over time, but it will not spoil.

SIMPLE STIR-FRY MARINADE

INGREDIENTS:

- Protein of choice
- 1 teaspoon of vegetable, peanut, or canola oil
- ¼ teaspoon of salt
- ½ teaspoon of soy sauce

- ¼ teaspoon of ground black or white pepper
- ¼ teaspoon of sugar
- ½ teaspoon of Shaoxing wine
- ½ teaspoon of cornstarch

DIRECTIONS:

1. Pour all the ingredients into a bowl and mix with your hands to coat the protein on all sides.
2. Cover it and refrigerate for 35 minutes before cooking.

SHIO KOJI MARINADE

INGREDIENTS:

- 1⅔ cups of rice koji (a type of fermented rice)
- 7 tablespoons of kosher salt
- 1⅔ cups of water

DIRECTIONS:

1. Mix the rice koji and salt in a container with a lid. Use your hands or a spoon to break up any clumps in the koji.
2. Add the water to the koji-salt mixture. Stir until you get a consistent mixture and the salt has completely dissolved. This should take only 30 seconds.
3. Put the lid on the container and let the mixture sit at room temperature. Over the next 7 to 10 days, stir the mixture once a day as it ferments.
4. While it ferments, the mixture will thicken and develop a sweet and savory smell.
5. Once the fermentation is complete, transfer the shio koji marinade to an airtight container and refrigerate it. It can be kept in the fridge for up to 10 months.

BARBECUE SAUCE

INGREDIENTS:

- 1 cup of chicken broth
- 1 small onion, grated
- ½ cup of ketchup
- 1 tablespoon of brown mustard
- 2 tablespoons of Worcestershire sauce
- 2 tablespoons of spice rub
- 2 teaspoons of hot sauce, plus extra if necessary
- 2 tablespoons of cider vinegar, plus extra if necessary
- 1 teaspoon of liquid smoke, such as Wright's (Optional)
- ¼ cup of dark molasses, plus extra if necessary

DIRECTIONS:

1. Put all the ingredients in a small pot on the griddle over medium-low heat.
2. Stir the ingredients together and let them simmer for about 15 minutes. The sauce should get thicker as it cooks.
3. Taste the sauce and add more molasses, vinegar, or hot sauce to adjust the flavor.
4. Once the sauce has cooled, it can be stored in the fridge for a few months.

WHITE BARBECUE SAUCE

INGREDIENTS:

- ½ cup of apple cider vinegar
- ¼ teaspoon of garlic powder
- 2 cups of mayonnaise
- 2 tablespoons of fresh lemon juice
- 2 teaspoons of prepared yellow mustard
- ¼ cup of prepared extra-hot horseradish
- 1 teaspoon of kosher salt
- ½ teaspoon of cayenne pepper
- 1½ teaspoons of freshly ground black pepper

DIRECTIONS:

1. Mix the mayonnaise, vinegar, horseradish, lemon juice, mustard, black pepper, salt, cayenne pepper, and garlic powder in a bowl.
2. Stir everything until you get a consistent paste.
3. Cover the bowl and put the sauce in the fridge until you're ready to use it.

JERK SEASONING RUB

INGREDIENTS:

- 3 tablespoons of dried thyme
- 1 tablespoon of dried rosemary
- 3 tablespoons of cracked black pepper
- 1 tablespoon of ground cinnamon
- 2 tablespoons of turbinado sugar
- 3 tablespoons of onion powder
- 1 tablespoon of cayenne pepper
- 2 tablespoons of garlic powder
- 1½ tablespoons of sea salt
- 1 tablespoon of ground ginger
- 3 tablespoons of ground allspice
- 1 tablespoon of dried sage
- 1 tablespoon of ground nutmeg
- 1 tablespoon of dried marjoram

DIRECTIONS:

1. Put all the ingredients in a bowl.
2. Use a whisk to mix the ingredients together until they are properly combined.
3. Spoon the finished seasoning rub into a glass jar with a tight-fitting lid. This will help keep the seasoning fresh for months.

ALL-STAR CHICKEN MARINADE

INGREDIENTS:

- ¾ cup of soy sauce
- ½ cup of red wine vinegar
- ½ cup of Worcestershire sauce
- 1½ cups of vegetable oil
- ⅓ cup of lemon juice
- 2 tablespoons of dry mustard
- 1 tablespoon of black pepper
- 1 teaspoon of salt
- 1½ teaspoons of minced fresh parsley

DIRECTIONS:

1. Mix the oil, soy sauce, Worcestershire sauce, vinegar, and lemon juice.
2. Stir in the dry mustard, salt, pepper, and parsley.
3. Use this marinade to coat the chicken pieces you want to cook. The longer you let the chicken sit in the marinade, the more flavor it will soak up.

PORK CHOP MARINADE

INGREDIENTS:

- ¼ cup of apple cider vinegar
- 2 tablespoons of grainy mustard
- ¼ cup of brown sugar
- ½ teaspoon of red pepper flakes
- ½ cup of olive oil
- 2 minced garlic cloves
- Salt and pepper for seasoning

DIRECTIONS:

1. Mix the olive oil, vinegar, brown sugar, mustard, minced garlic, and red pepper flakes in a large bowl.
2. Season the marinade with as much salt and pepper as you like.
3. Place the pork chops in the bowl, and make sure they are fully coated with the marinade.
4. Cover the bowl and put it in the fridge for at least 2 hours before you cook the pork chops.

MEXICAN MARINADE

INGREDIENTS:

- ⅓ cup of white vinegar
- ⅓ cup of cider vinegar
- Juice from 1 lime
- ⅓ cup of olive oil
- 6 minced garlic cloves

- 1 tablespoon of dried oregano
- 2 tablespoons of ground cumin
- ⅓ cup of fresh cilantro, chopped
- 1 tablespoon of whole black peppercorns
- 1 teaspoon of salt

DIRECTIONS:

1. Put all the ingredients in a bowl and stir them well.
2. For the best flavor, making this marinade a day ahead is a good idea so the flavors can blend properly.
3. Place the meat you want to marinate in a container and pour the marinade over it. Let it sit in the marinade for at least 6 hours before cooking.

- **Vegetables:** Dice any leftover vegetables like onions, peppers, mushrooms, etc., and sauté them until they caramelize. You can then use them as a topping for burgers, tacos, omelets, or even mix them into a hash.

- **Proteins:** If you have any leftover cooked meats, like chicken, steak, or pork, you can quickly reheat them on the griddle. Then you can use that meat to make quesadillas, tacos, or breakfast burritos. Or you could always make sliced pork tenderloin or salmon filets and serve them over a salad or in a sandwich.

- **Grains:** For leftover grains like rice, quinoa, or farro, you can make delicious griddle cakes or fritters. Just mix the grains with some beaten eggs, herbs, and spices, then cook them on the flat top like pancakes. You can also use your leftover grains to make a tasty fried rice; just add vegetables, protein, and a sauce.

- **Bread or tortilla:** Make some mini griddle-cooked pizza bites by topping bread/tortilla rounds with sauce, cheese, and toppings. Or turn stale bread into homemade croutons by cubing it and crisping it on your griddle. You can even use the griddle to make churro-inspired treats by cooking strips of dough and coating them in cinnamon sugar.

Conclusion

The gas griddle has proven itself to be an indispensable tool in the modern home kitchen, offering unparalleled versatility, convenience, and ease of use. It is no one-trick pony. You have seen the true breadth of what this simple yet remarkable appliance can do. There's a certain joy and satisfaction that comes from cooking on a griddle—the sights, the sounds, the smells that fill the kitchen. It's almost meditative when you stand before that heated surface, tending to your food with a spatula in your hand. You feel connected to the most fundamental pleasures of home cooking in a way that surpasses simply producing a finished meal.

Of course, the real proof is in the pudding (or the pancakes, as it were). The gas griddle has repeatedly shown that it can and will deliver five-star-level results right at home. Those golden-brown sears, that perfect, even cooking—it's the kind of quality that has to be experienced to be fully appreciated.

As you've worked your way through this cookbook, the hope is that you've not only learned the techniques and discovered new favorite recipes but also felt the pull to experiment, improvise, and make the gas griddle your own. After all, what is cooking if not a process of discovery—trying new flavor combinations, advancing your skills, and putting your own stamp on every recipe?

No matter what recipes you choose to try, remember to have fun with it. Cooking should be a joyful, liberating experience, not a rigid set of rules to be followed. So don't be worried about things getting a little out of hand or trying things that might not work the first time. The more you play and explore, the more you'll learn about your tastes, skills, and cooking style. Some of the best meals were born from happy accidents and inspired improvisations. The only limits are the ones you place on yourself.

References

Abonour, R. (2023, July 28). *19 Grilled Burger Recipes to Make All Summer Long.* Serious Eats. https://www.seriouseats.com/burger-recipes

Evinks, the. (2023, October 30). *Blackstone Pizza.* Gimme Some Grilling. https://gimmesomegrilling.com/blackstone-pizza/

Filson, M. (2022, November 30). *75 Homemade Pizza Recipes That Ended Our Love Affair with Takeout.* Delish. https://www.delish.com/cooking/recipe-ideas/g269/homemade-pizza-recipes/?slide=1

Jaramillo, C. (2022, June 7). *Vegan Recipes for the Grill.* Grillio. https://grillio.com/blog/vegan-grill-recipes/

Jeanie, & Jack. (2020, May 28). *Homemade Pita Bread.* Love and Lemons. https://www.loveandlemons.com/pita-bread-recipe/#wprm-recipe-container-48019

Koncker, C. (2021, July 16). *Spinach Feta Quesadilla.* Midwexican. https://www.midwexican.com/spinach-feta-quesadilla/

Lowder, C. (2021, February 19). *Easy Pasta Recipes for Deliciously Fuss-Free Dinners.* Delish. https://www.delish.com/cooking/recipe-ideas/g3176/weeknight-pasta-dinners/

Megan, & Michael. (2024, February 5). *29 Blackstone Recipes Perfect for Outdoor Cooking.* Fresh off the Grid. https://www.freshoffthegrid.com/blackstone-recipes/

Michel, C. (2024, June 11). *You Can Make These Dinner Recipes in 30 Minutes or Less.* Country Living. https://www.countryliving.com/food-drinks/g648/quick-easy-dinner-recipes/

MS, L. E. (2020, June 29). *Best Summer Grill Recipes: All Plant-Based.* Forks over Knives. https://www.forksoverknives.com/recipes/vegan-menus-collections/best-summer-grill-recipes-all-plant-based/

Murray, T. (2023, July 20). *30 Easy Flatbread Recipes and Topping Ideas That Are Even Better than Pizza.* Food Network. https://www.foodnetwork.com/recipes/photos/flatbread-recipe-ideas

Neal. (2023, June 2). *Cooking Burgers on the Griddle - 8 Griddle Burger Recipes to Try!* The Flat Top King. https://theflattopking.com/griddle-burgers/

Nisha. (2022, June 7). *Black Bean Quesadillas with Corn (No Cook).* Honey, Whats Cooking. https:/www. honeywhatscooking.com/black-bean-and-corn-quesadillas/

Ronning, S. (2024, March 6). *Blackstone griddle sandwich recipes.* From Michigan to the Table. https:/ frommichigantothetable.com/griddle-sandwich-recipes/

Stanko, C. (2024, May 9). *35 Char Grilled Appetizer Recipes.* Taste of Home. https:/www.tasteofhome.com/ collection/grilled-appetizer-recipes/

Made in United States
Orlando, FL
24 May 2025